Riptides
& Solaces Unforeseen

RIPTIDES
& Solaces Unforeseen

A MEMOIR

Debby Mayer

Epigraph Books
Rhinebeck, New York

Heartfelt thanks to my dear friends who patiently read this manuscript and gave me feedback on it, and special thanks to Linda Mattis, who has been there since the beginning.

Book design: Bill McAllister

Library of Congress Control Number: 2021922984
ISBN: 978-1-936940-51-6
Epigraph Books
22 East Market Street Suite 304
Rhinebeck, NY 12572

Printed in the United States of America

For Dan Zinkus

The Run

"They didn't hurt," Dan says about his legs. "They just didn't move."

It's Monday, May 6, and Dan takes his usual run around the closed landfill two-tenths of a mile from our house. It's circled by a dirt maintenance road that's exactly a mile long—he measured it on his car's odometer—and he customarily makes three or four circuits, running between a seven- and an eight-minute mile. He's 55 years old, 6 feet tall, and weighs 170 pounds. He's been running between four and six days a week since his 30th birthday. The previous winter was mild and dry; he didn't have to cut back much.

On May 6, he has a terrible run. "3x," he notes on his daily calendar; "40m [minutes], dead legs." It's bad enough so that he calls me at my office. "They didn't hurt," he says about his legs, "they just didn't move."

Dan, who works at home, often calls me with one health complaint or another, none of which I can do anything about from my desk in the publications office of a college half an hour south of our house. His back hurts, or his stomach, or the inside of his knee. Few, if any, of these complaints drive him to a doctor; rather, he calls me at work, and I try to suggest what might be wrong.

This time I do sympathize. After living with him for 24 years, I still love him dearly, passionately. I want him to be healthy and happy, and running is important to him. He's complained recently about slow runs—the previous week he had done only a nine-minute mile, which is more my speed—but what he describes today is new.

We go out that night to the movies, as we often do. We see *Nine Queens*, an Argentinean film about con men. Clever but unfair, I tell Dan afterward; the set-up takes place long before the opening scene. He dismisses this with a shrug, as he does a lot of what I say these days, and I'm a little bit hurt, but the film stays with me.

"Altered reality," says my friend Margaret in a phone conversation the next day. "It's disturbing."

Exactly. Because we've been talking about Dan, too. "He seemed so quiet at dinner Saturday," says Margaret.

"—He's been having these oddly slow runs . . . "

Dan holds off running on Tuesday, and as we eat supper that night he says something about seeing a sports doctor. When my reaction to that idea apparently isn't warm enough, he says, "Well, what do you think I should do?"

"—I think you should see a neurologist," I say, surprising myself.

"A neurologist!" He packs disbelief and scorn into one word.

"—We know it's not a sports injury. You'll waste two weeks getting an appointment with a sports doctor, and then he'll tell you everything is fine. It sounds systemic."

"—I'll call Hahn," he says.

"Good idea." As usual, Dan is right. I've jumped a step; better to see our family doctor first, someone who knows him and can look at the whole picture.

Dr. Hahn fits Dan in the next day, Wednesday the 8th, and I'm glad. "Tell him I think your speech is getting slurred."

Dan gives me a look that says he will tell Hahn no such thing.

I have an appointment that day with the optometrist in the building next door to Dr. Hahn's office, and when I come out, Dan lopes over with our two basenjis, Cooper and Lulu. He takes the dogs—small, shorthaired hounds that don't bark—along for the ride whenever he can. His gait makes me uneasy; I'm used to his striding, not loping.

"He doesn't know what's wrong with me," he says, and we both laugh. Dr. Hahn often confesses puzzlement over our ailments. He's declared Dan basically fit and told him to keep running. He ordered some blood work through the lab in his building and left for a week's vacation.

At supper Dan reports further. "He asked me if I was depressed. I said no."

"You said *what*!"

"Well, I'm not as depressed as I was."

When I tell this to Margaret, she guffaws. "I'm sorry," she says immediately, "I know it's not funny."

But it is funny, and that's why I told her: our clever, articulate Dan avoids an honest answer by telling the absolute truth.

Thursday dawns rainy, so Dan takes another day off, but Friday is nice enough, and he sets out before breakfast. I'm aware of being alone for a while as I fix our breakfasts, keeping an eye on the clock because my office sets great store on punctuality. Finally I set his tea steeping—he switched to green tea this year, for the antioxidants—and sit down with my cereal and coffee.

I'm about halfway through this repast when he arrives at the sliding door between the back deck and the kitchen. His scowl is fierce.

"You started breakfast without me!"

Looking back, there were signs.

Again, he was right—for two-dozen years we'd eaten breakfast together. We might each dive into our favorite section of the newspaper, but it was a communal activity, and neither of us started before we were both seated. Until this past winter, when he stopped waiting for me.

I had teased him in the past about becoming a curmudgeon as he grew older, but over the winter he had become downright unpleasant. Since we lived in a rural county in upstate New York, and since he worked at home as a freelance book editor, a lot of his grouchiness fell on me: impatience when I couldn't break up the dog biscuits fast enough, anger one Saturday when I bought AA batteries instead of the AAA that he wanted; fury, on one of our last trips to New York, when I had only a token in a subway station that took only MetroCards.

But it wasn't just me. In Hudson, our "city," fifteen minutes west, he got into a fight with another driver over a parking place. Where anyone else would have let the man have his stupid space, Dan held out, sitting in the car with the dogs, throwing some change at the man so he could pay for a meter somewhere else, and the man saying that was assault, he was going to call the cops, and my thinking that Dan could have wound up in the newspaper police blotter and it would have served him right.

People later admitted to finding him "off" that winter and spring. "He didn't seem to hold his liquor as well," said Paul, one of his closest friends. "I thought it was our age."

"Just not his usual attention to detail," said Owen, a coworker at *Time*. "We wondered if he had a health problem."

"Just moving slower," said our 81-year-old plumber.

Dan had suffered from depression periodically for as long as I had known him, and I thought this was one of those times. Walking the dogs in Hudson one Saturday, we passed the office of a man whose shingle said he was a psychotherapist. "There's somebody I could see," said Dan, apropos of nothing.

"Would you really see that therapist in Hudson?" I asked later, at home.

"No," he said, dismissive again. "I don't even know who he is."

I remember thinking, if he won't see someone, then I will. One of us has to. My church offered a counseling service; I could start there. I didn't know who the counselor was and I frankly didn't care.

Still, I put it off. My complaints were details, I told myself, in a life that had altered only slightly and might yet readjust again with spring. Our house was small—1,100 square feet if you counted every inch—and every winter I found myself checking the local real estate magazines, looking for a new home for us, one whose sole requirement was to let me escape from the sound of the television.

Spring, which pushed us both outdoors, always cheered us up. We spread out onto the screened-in porch. Dan set up his outdoor shower on the deck. I would realize that nothing we could afford would give us the land and privacy we had now.

On May 4, my church in Hudson celebrated its bicentennial with a special Eucharist and a reception under a tent on the courthouse lawn across the street.

The bishop came down from Albany, and a bevy of priests celebrated the Mass in full regalia. The church, which seats 200, was almost full, and everyone acted as if my publicizing the event had performed this miracle. I read the Old Testament lesson, which was from Genesis ("I shall be with you to protect you wherever you go," God tells Jacob), and our rector emeritus said he heard it that afternoon as he never had before. The sky was cloudless, the air sweet with the promise of spring.

"Perfect!" I wrote in my daybook.

I meant the day, of course, the moment. I knew my life wasn't perfect—in an undercurrent something was askew, something more than my disappointment that Dan would set foot in church only on Christmas Eve. But no one's life was perfect, and mine was good.

Still, some days that spring I didn't look forward to coming home.

And some days that spring I was frightened. The time when I could not understand what he was saying, even from context. The rainy Saturday afternoon when, returning from errands, I found that he had left our old Honda in the driveway with its lights on. I stopped immediately and turned off the Honda lights, before I parked my Jetta.

"What were you doing out there?" he asked.

I kept my tone matter-of-fact, even though he would have scorned me for such an oversight.

He thought about it. "It's OK," he said. "I only drove it a little ways with the lights on."

And the last weekend we spent in New York, in April—was it walking to the Chinese restaurant, or to the Museum of Modern Art—when I said to him, "Do you realize I'm walking faster than you?"

He shrugged, but I was unnerved; I had spent 25 years trying to keep up with him.

On May 10, Dan's run has been dreadful. In 40 minutes he's been able to circle the landfill only three times, or three miles. Again, his legs don't hurt; they just don't work.

But it doesn't occur to me to call Hahn's office, find out who's covering for him, and try to get the blood work results from that doctor. Partly because I still have no sense of emergency, and partly because I know, in my heart of hearts, the blood work will be inconclusive.

Instead, we live our life. Friday night we go to the movies again. In the car we talk about Dan's phone conversation that day with Paul. Unbidden, Paul had told him his speech was slurred.

"There you are," I say. "The two people who know you best." Dan is driving; I'm speaking to his profile in the twilight. He's one of those men whose looks have improved with age: his beard and what's left of his hair, gone gray, soften his face without weakening it; his modified aviator glasses look better than any previous style.

"He said maybe I have Parkinson's."

"I was trying to think of something that he might be able to function with," Paul says later. "He was furious when I told him his speech was slurred. He said, 'What did you do, talk to Debby?'"

Parkinson's; the best of a bad lot. Michael J. Fox. Dan has looked it up on the Web, and that's all I want to do, too, tell him to turn the car around, drive me home so I can get in front of my computer. I don't; his search was inconclusive—he doesn't have any palsy—and my hysteria won't help.

Saturday . . . 44 degrees, clear, Dan notes in his calendar, 7:30 a.m. (a late rising for him). He keeps his calendar daily, recording the weather morning and night, his exercise, and a brief recap of the day's events. This Saturday he writes nothing more.

When I start his tea water, he says, "I'll have coffee," and I feel like we've turned a corner, into a life in which antioxidants don't matter, a life in which you can do whatever you want because . . . why not?

Dan and the dogs meet me in Hudson after my church vestry meeting. We shop for plants, buy rhubarb pie at a library bake sale. We're in two cars, and I'm uneasy. "It doesn't seem to affect my driving," he says, but I don't see how it can't.

Matt and Julie call from Bremerton, Washington, to firm up plans for their trip east in early June. For the first time ever, Dan doesn't pick up the other phone, but I don't say anything about his health. We're one of three stops on their trip; they might as well come, and see what there is to see.

Sunday, Mother's Day, we treat my mother and stepfather and Dan's mother and sister to brunch. The talk is of gardens and movies; the two mothers exchange news of ailments.

"Is Dan all right?" my mother asks later, when she calls to thank me. "He seemed so quiet."

"He's fine," I say, "the restaurant was noisy," half of which is true. He's afraid people will find his speech slurred, I'm sure, but to tell my mother Dan's problems and my unsubstantiated fears would result in hourly phone calls with questions I couldn't answer, urgings I couldn't tolerate.

As I leave for the office on Monday, Dan gives me an order, quiet, but not casual: "Ask Susan if she knows a neurologist." Susan and her husband, Ed, are old friends; he's a doctor and she's a nurse practitioner, who heads the Student Health Service at the college where I work.

First I Google "Parkinson's Disease," and yes, ancillary symptoms include slurred speech and difficulty walking. But he doesn't have the main symptom, palsy.

Then I e-mail Susan. I mention our lunch in the faculty dining room last week and say, "if you get your walking group organized, let me know," and then, "Can you or Ed suggest a neurologist? . . . This is a matter of some importance."

"We both really like a group practice in Kingston," Susan writes back an hour later. "This practice has an excellent reputation among doctors in this area. They are considered top rate." She names three of the doctors she knows and adds, "There is a woman in the practice that I've heard is really good. I don't know her name." She gives me their phone number. "I hope this is helpful."

Monday night as I'm washing the dishes, the words *brain tumor* fall into my mind. I stop, frozen in mid-swipe. I see myself take off the rubber gloves, walk to the computer in Dan's office alcove off the living room, and run those two words on Google.

I don't do it. He's lying on the living room floor, his head propped on a sofa pillow, trying to read. The dogs are stretched along his legs like two small fawns. What are you doing? he would say. *Brain tumor!* he would say. As if I had accused him of something.

Tuesday Dan takes a walk around the landfill, in an effort to get some exercise. At the office I Google "brain tumor," go directly to "symptoms," then wend my way through the multitudes of brain tumors. Most of them result in excruciating headaches, one of the few health problems Dan has never complained of. Finally, I find one that causes slurred speech, vision problems—he's been seeing an ophthalmologist and putting prescription eye drops in his eyes every night for months—and movement difficulties. And it's operable.

Wednesday Dr. Hahn returns from his vacation. The blood work shows a possible anemia, but nothing that would result in slurred speech and the inability to run. He schedules Dan for an MRI on Friday.

I pick up my new glasses and wearing them, I can hardly see. I've gone for progressives, which allow me to pick out every leaf on the new dogwood outside my office window but not to find a comfortable position for computer work, playing the piano, reading—things I do every day.

Dan and I meet at a kitchen center near my office with the man who's been doing a computer redesign of our kitchen. Afterward Dan wants to have lunch at Gigi's, a trattoria that's his favorite restaurant of the moment. I've already been gone from the office for an hour, and Gigi's can be slow, but I meet him there anyway. The place and its food make him happy, and what if . . . *what if* happens?

It's the last time we eat there.

Thursday Dan and the dogs come to my office around four, but I can't get away early, so he takes them for a walk. The campus is on the Hudson River, and part of it is a mansion with an Italianate garden in full spring bloom. When they return at five I can see dirt on the front of his shirt. "I fell three times," he whispers.

"Take it easy!" I whisper back, feeling my eyes go wide. I have no other advice, and no consolation. *"Take it easy."*

Thursday is dog agility night in our household, at a ring between my office and our house. Agility training lets dogs do what they like to do anyway—jump and climb and run around. In her second summer of training, two-year-old Lulu is getting good at it; Dan takes her to an extra, private lesson on Wednesday mornings. Thursday evenings are for all of us. I sit with Cooper, who at 15 is quite blind and no longer able to trot the course, and Dan runs around with Lulu.

"Let me take her tonight," I say as we arrive at the ring.

He doesn't acknowledge me, and he falls on their first time around the course, a fairly spectacular fall, head over heels, losing both the dog and his glasses. Then we switch.

I've arranged to take Friday morning off to go with Dan to the imaging center in Hudson. I hadn't thought my presence would really be necessary—"I'll just hold your foot," I told him—but by Friday his gait is so unsteady he clearly can't drive.

"Look at my handwriting," he says in the waiting room. It's barely legible.

I put my arm around his waist. "You're getting this test. We'll find out what's wrong."

I finish filling out the forms for him and take them up to the receptionist. "You will be faxing an initial report to Dr. Hahn this morning." I say it calmly, with a smile, but I don't let myself make it a question.

"Oh no, dear," she says. "It takes three business days to get a reading."

I almost swoon. But having a hysterical fit in this small, windowless waiting room, before a receptionist who doesn't set policy, won't help. I have to think of something else.

The technician is a slim, pleasant strawberry blond. She explains the process to us carefully. It will be long—Dr. Hahn has ordered a full series. It will be noisy. Dan must lie perfectly still on the narrow bed that will be slid into the huge imaging machine, a sort of iron lung on steroids. She will cover his eyes, but if he feels claustrophobic, he can signal her and she'll let him out. He can have a sedative, if he wants.

She leaves the room and reappears behind a window. I kiss his lips and sit on a chair at his feet. The bed slides into the machine, leaving Dan visible from the knees down. I don't hold his foot, for fear of making him start.

The first series of images takes about 40 minutes, and never have I been wrapped in such astonishing noise. We're not inside a ship's engine room, we're inside the engine; I can feel my bones vibrate. I close my eyes against it.

Three years ago I spent a week in Columbia Memorial Hospital here in Hudson, having my blood thinned against a deep vein thrombosis. Dan visited me twice a day every day, wearing a different one of his Hawaiian "vacation man" shirts each time "to cheer you up." I signed a Health Care Proxy, so if a scheduled test hadn't been given, he found out why not. If it had been given, he got the results. Articulate and fast on his feet—everything I am not—he took care of my care.

The technician gives him a break. We all chat; he says he's fine. She slides him back in for a different series. This time I sit with her in the relative quiet of the control room. We continue talking; it turns out that we live in the same town and have mutual friends, including Susan and Ed.

"You know," I say, looking toward her notes on the console, "Dan didn't give you all his symptoms." All he has written down is "can't run."

"What else?" she says, picking up a pen, and I tick off the lengthening list. From there I move on to how this has been going on for two weeks, the doctor was on vacation; really, Dan should have had this MRI a week ago, and Dr. Hahn's office closes at 1 p.m. on Fridays.

She nods. "When we're done, I'll walk the film over to the radiologist. He can phone a report to Dr. Hahn."

"Thank you," I say, my gratitude heartfelt, eternal.

As for Dan, he's hungry and wants to have lunch at another of his favorite restaurants, the Red Barn. Again I'm due back at work, but again it's lunchtime and I feel as if I have just jumped a set of hurdles and I am incapable of saying no, I can't eat lunch with you, to my lover who is deteriorating before my eyes.

We eat succulent soft-shell crab sandwiches, and when we get home we have missed a call from Dr. Hahn. Dan shrugs, but I listen to the message twice, furious with myself for not coming straight home. An initial reading shows a disturbance in the brain cells at the back of the neck, he says. Unfortunately, he's going away for the weekend, he adds with a little laugh, but he will leave some sample packets of medication for Dan at the blood lab in his building, and "if you feel worse, go to the hospital."

I tear down to the lab, pick up the pills, then go to my office. At home that evening Dan opens the package and reads the accompanying pamphlet, as he always does with medication. This is Pletal, for people who have pain in their legs after exercise. The pamphlet is all about a narrowing of the arteries that decreases blood flow to the legs and thus oxygen to the leg muscles. Pletal's effect is to dilate arteries supplying blood to the legs.

Dan and I stare at each other. We're sitting at the large oval table in our dining area off the kitchen, me at the head of it, Dan to my right, so that we both have a view of the yard through the sliding glass door. We're sitting in a home we've owned for eighteen years, two miles from the post office, five miles from the nearest store. We have neighbors, but we can't see their houses from ours. We chose this place, "centrally located in the middle of nowhere," as Dan says, and this life. We're accustomed to taking care of ourselves. But this, this is more than solitude and independence. This is swept away by a riptide into new territory, without a guide or a net.

Dan takes the pills anyway. And when we go food shopping the next morning, Saturday, he won't let me buy grapefruit juice, because the pamphlet says not to take Pletal with grapefruit juice.

We've stopped at the imaging center to pick up his MRI film on the way to the market, and I've left him in the car, looking at it. So I'm startled—and frightened—to see him coming toward me in his new walk, his body lurching forward at a 45-degree angle, step by sliding step. I give him the cart to push, and he hangs onto it. Always interested in new products, he has me buy some tuna that comes in a sealed pouch instead of a can.

At home we have a message from a Dr. Ruggieri, who's covering this weekend for Dr. Hahn. Additional blood tests have found no problems. He leaves the number of his service. I put away the food and make sandwiches for us while Dan stretches out on the bed with the dogs, Cooper alongside him, Lulu on top of his legs.

He eats his sandwich, but when I collect the plate he says his head aches. He feels worse than yesterday.

I sit down on the edge of the bed, part of me terrified, part of me thinking that this is probably the hypochondria kicking in, and *I should use it.* "Let me call this doctor, see if he has any ideas."

I leave word with Dr. Ruggieri's service, and from that moment, I use my given name. Prior to that, never mind my age, I had always been Debby. I knew it was a child's name, but I liked it, and it was what I had always gone by, what I had put on the covers of two books. Now, to the medical establishment, I am Deborah, and he is Daniel. We are adults, we have names. "This is Deborah Mayer. I'm calling on behalf of Daniel Zinkus." I must have said it a hundred times in the next one hundred days.

When Dr. Ruggieri calls back, I speak to him. Without asking, I know that Dan cannot manage a coherent telephone conversation with a doctor. I describe his symptoms, adding the headache.

He should see a neurologist sooner, rather than later, says Dr. Ruggieri. He could admit Dan to Columbia Memorial today, but there will be no neurologist on duty until Monday. We could go to Kingston Hospital, forty-five minutes southwest of us, where someone from Kingston Neurology will see Dan today, or to Albany Medical Center, an hour north, where there will also be a neurologist on duty.

Dan and I decide to call Kingston Neurology. I leave our number with their service, and Dr. Alma Singh calls back. She listens, asks questions. "If you want to come down here, I'll see him," she says. "Or, you could go to Albany Medical Center."

AMC is probably the best of the three hospitals, but neither of us wants to go there, picturing a Saturday emergency room straight out of *ER*, full of wailing victims, without a doctor who has time for us. Dan wants to go to

Columbia Memorial tomorrow, and wait one day to see a neurologist. It's tempting—he'd be safe and in Hudson, only fifteen minutes away. When I had my blood thinned there it seemed perfectly good.

But "Dr. Ruggieri said you should see a neurologist sooner, rather than later." It's May 18, only twelve days after his bad run, and he can hardly walk. In Kingston, which is near my office, we have a neurologist, someone Susan and Ed recommend. Dan agrees to see her that afternoon. I pack a bag for him, in case they admit him, including his MRI film, *Pillar of Fire*, which he's been reading, and the CD player he gave me when I was in the hospital. I choose some CDs—an Ian Tyson album, Bach suites for cello, *Follies*, an anthology of arias sung by Callas, and the sound track from *O Brother Where Art Thou*. I call Dr. Singh to tell her we're coming, and she gives me precise directions to the hospital, which Dan renders useless by having me drive to Kingston on an entirely different route. But his sense of direction is still infallible.

Kingston

"Are you on any medication?"

Dr. Alma Singh is small and slim, somewhere between 35 and 45. In a glistening white examining room with four empty beds she has Dan follow her pen with his eyes. She taps his knee with a little hammer that she carries in a leather case. She watches him walk the length of the room and back. She asks if he is on any medication, and we show her the Pletal. She shakes her head, wrinkling her little nose. She takes the MRI film away to review it.

"What do you think?" I ask Dan.

"Seems all right," he says, which matches my assessment. Do a pen and a hammer report the vast change that's taking place in him? Is she noncommittal because she doesn't want to frighten us?

I follow signs through a quiet hallway to the washroom. On my way back I run into Dr. Singh, chewing on something as she walks.

She swallows. "Sorry, birthday party." It's 4:30 and she probably hasn't had lunch, so I hold my tongue and don't say please, no frosting on Dan's film.

Still later, she comes back to us. "All right," she says, "I'm going to admit him. I can't tell you what's wrong based on that MRI—we may have to do another." A neurosurgeon will see him, maybe this evening, for sure tomorrow.

There will be another wait before Dan's assigned a room, so we agree I should go home. I kiss him and try to hold him for a moment.

"Give me the cell phone," he says.

I leave him in the eerily quiet hospital in dingy downtown Kingston, telling myself we've made the right move. They will examine him. They will tell us something. The New York State Thruway is damp and slick, crowded with trucks. She doesn't know what's wrong with him. The MRI isn't clear. I cross the Rip Van Winkle Bridge, back onto our side of the Hudson River; home safe, but alone.

I keep to our routine, walking the dogs, feeding them, measuring the rain in the gauge—a little over an inch, good—and recording it on Dan's calendar.

He calls: he has a room, but he got in too late for dinner.

He calls again: they've brought him cookies and milk.

I don't feel like playing the piano, but I do. I take a weekly lesson and the studio's annual concert is set for June 12, less than a month away. My three short pieces—a Bach prelude, Philip Glass's Metamorphosis 3, and Kid Ory's "Get Out of Here"—are almost ready. But I play badly tonight, missing chords and combinations I know by heart. My new glasses are driving me nuts; I can see the top measure of notes only by craning my neck. I tell myself it's been worthwhile just to try to keep the pieces in my fingers.

I don't play the piano again until October.

Sunday I find two *New York Times* crossword puzzles in a pile of newspapers on Dan's desk. He's started Thursday's but hasn't touched Friday's. He does the *Times* puzzle every day, in ink, in about 10 minutes. I bring the puzzles with me to the hospital.

"Do you want these? You haven't done them."

He's alone in a large, two-person room, sitting on the bed in his gray sweat suit. He accepts the puzzles, but what he wants to do is go downstairs to the cafeteria and get a cup of tea. He probably isn't allowed off the floor, but no one's paying any attention to us, and I'll take care of him. We ride the elevator down to the basement cafeteria, a windowless place made drearier by crayoned messages signed with smiley faces. We buy mugs of tea and packages of cookies. "Let me carry yours," I say, but he doesn't acknowledge me and lurches to a table, splattering tea in great puddles with every step. I follow with paper napkins, wiping up.

He's sipping his tea, his back to the drying floor, when I sit down. "Can't talk about my condition," he says, tapping a laminated sign on the table.

"Or mine. What else is new?"

The neurosurgeon examined him.

"Good. What's he like?"

"He's all right."

Next we explore the first floor of the hospital, wrapped together, my arm around his waist, his on my shoulders. We find the gift shop and browse through its newspapers and magazines. Dan wants to step outdoors, and I'm relieved when a security guard stops us. We go back to his room the long way, without passing the nurse's station.

Monday I go to the hospital at lunchtime to find they've installed a belt on his bed that beeps when he gets up.

"I found him getting off the elevator this morning!" says the nurse. Tall, gray-haired, she is unique among nurses today in that she wears her cap: two starched white wings soar from either side of her head.

"He was probably just looking for a *Times*," I say, swallowing a giggle.

He was. He had put a dollar into the pocket of his gray sweat suit and gone in search of a paper. Now he is not to leave his bed unaided.

"She can't keep me here," Dan says, with an odd, crafty smile.

"And who's gonna drive you home."

He looks away.

"What's this?" On a rolling tray is a straw basket filled with houseplants—African violet, ivy, geranium, sedum. They're from Sonia, his former business partner.

"She called me last night," I say. "She's horrified that they haven't started an IV in you. She kept saying, 'My mother's an RN, she says they should have started an IV right away.' I said, 'He's eating food, why should they start an IV?'"

Dan nods, sympathetic. In the '80s he and Sonia ran a textbook packaging house. She still calls him daily, seeking advice on one matter or another—a book project, her trip to Nepal, the climbing wall in her backyard.

The hospital continues testing him—spinal tap, urinalysis, chest X-ray, extensive blood work—but Dr. Singh has already started him on steroids. She's not sure of a diagnosis, but it may be multiple sclerosis, and if it is, the steroids should help quickly.

I report this to my coworkers after lunch. Elliot, my immediate supervisor, is scornful. "That's what they say when they can't think of anything else."

He might as well have slapped me.

"Men!" sighs Mike, my officemate. "They never say anything right."

True. I suck in my tears and Google multiple sclerosis . . . more frequently seen in women . . . usually comes on slowly. But not impossible here.

"If Dan were a docile patient, then we'd worry," says Margaret on the phone that night. I try to laugh, but I am worried. I wish he would stay in bed, do what they tell him, give them honest answers. He seems, in some odd way, not to be taking this seriously.

My call list of friends—no family yet, not till I know more—is growing. Sonia. Margaret. Paul. Linda.

I've started taking Lulu to my dog-friendly office, so that she won't have to stay in her crate for nine hours. Dan would never crate Cooper, so I leave him home, and on Monday I ask Linda if instead of meeting me for lunch, would she stop by the house and let Cooper out.

Linda enters the yard through the back gate off the driveway. She opens the sliding glass door that gives out onto the deck and the fenced-in yard and calls to Cooper. He comes to the door, but he won't step outside. Linda sits in a wooden rocker on the deck and talks to him gently. She tells him about Dan and Lulu and me, and why he should come out. Cooper sits just inside the open door, his eyes cloudy with cataracts, his fox-like head cocked slightly, listening with his selectively deaf hearing. He will be 16 next month, and he has always had a job to do at home. *Watch the house!* we say when we go out. *Watch the house!* He can't watch the house if he lets some woman he barely knows coax him out of it. After ten minutes, Linda closes the door and leaves.

Tuesday when I arrive at the hospital, Dan's in a different room, right across from the nurse's station. They've decided to do another full-scale brain MRI, with and without contrast, and another spinal tap, with contrast. They've also done a CAT scan of his head, because he fell out of bed onto it. They're continuing the steroids every eight hours, though he shows no sign of responding to them. While I'm there, he decides to listen to some music, and puts on his earphones. He stares straight ahead, a half-smile of contentment on his face, like a man who is alone.

Since Monday, the target date for his discharge has been Wednesday. Dr. Singh started the steroids with that in mind and now, even with no response, she plans to finish the testing and let him go. "His insurance is already saying that he could have these tests as an outpatient," she tells me.

Dan wants to go home. I feel cowardly and unloving to object, but what am I supposed to do with him? Wednesday morning Dr. Singh's office leaves a message on my voicemail at work: she will be discharging Dan at lunchtime so that I can pick him up, and she has been in contact with a neurosurgeon in Albany that we are to see.

I misunderstand the message. I think I am to pick up Dan in Kingston and drive him an hour north to Albany, where we have an appointment with a doctor. That's what I tell Elliot when I leave the office.

What we actually have is a referral to a neurosurgeon, who might want to do a brain biopsy; I am to call his office and make an appointment with him.

Dr. Singh still doesn't know what's wrong with Dan. All the tests have been negative or inconclusive. It's not

Lyme, and it's probably not multiple sclerosis, but there is still one MS test result pending. We might get that result before the long Memorial Day weekend coming up, or we might not. She can't make a diagnosis from the latest MRI. It shows a problem with the brain cells at the back of the neck, but not the cause. We're to take the film and show it to the neurosurgeon.

I repack Dan's suitcase. He's half-dressed, in his own shirt and hospital pajama bottoms, because he has become incontinent. A portable plastic urinal is hooked to his bed rail; another lies on a tray table, still sealed in a plastic bag. Dan and I are backpackers, on whom nothing is wasted; I tuck the sealed urinal into the suitcase.

I find the two *New York Times* puzzles from last week, untouched, and throw them away, embarrassed by my insensitivity at bringing them. Then I wait. He's insisting on finishing his lunch—"I paid for this"—his eyes glued to the TV screen.

Dr. Singh comes by to debrief us. She says Dan can drink, which surprises me, and only when I ask does she say, no, he should not drive. Dan scowls. The doctor writes out two prescriptions—one for a walker, the other for physical therapy.

And then she discharges him. She doesn't know what's wrong with him, and his condition has deteriorated for five days—now he's incontinent, unable to walk without help, and barely able to talk. A physical therapist—a quietly professional woman who is obviously disturbed that she has so little time with him—gives him fifteen minutes' training on a practice walker. We sign papers that say we agree with the discharge, that Dan is not being forced out of the hospital too soon.

I should have refused to sign. I should have sat down and crossed my arms and demanded a transfer to Albany Medical Center. But Dan wanted so badly to go home, and I thought we had a doctor.

Home

Our house has no hallways; except for the bathroom and the bedroom, each room gives onto the next without the formality of a door. The front door opens into the living room. To the left is the alcove Dan uses for his office; off that, the bathroom. At the far end of the living room is our bedroom, which ends with a sliding glass door into a screened-in porch. A doorway on the left wall of the living room is open to the kitchen, which opens onto a large dining area with a table that sits six (twelve, one night when we squeezed in) and, against one wall, my upright piano. A staircase in back of Dan's desk leads up to my study, a larger room we use as a guest room, and attic space behind a door that Dan painted yellow with a frame of marine blue. All the trim colors—the blue, the tomato, the upstairs bookcase painted in fuchsia—we found in a book called *Living Maya*. If the house could not be elegant, we said, it could be pretty.

There are two steps up to the back door or three up to the front; first then, the walker. Dan's face signals disagreement, but I drive on. Lulu burbles all over him, ecstatic. The day has become warm and he fiddles with the buttons for the automatic windows. Glancing into the rearview mirror I see that the back window on the other side of the car is all the way open, with cowgirl Lulu hanging out of it, a big hound grin on her face.

"Lulu, come!" The hysteria in my voice betrays me as I reach backwards for her with my right arm while I steer with my left hand, downtown in a city I don't know, as Dan pushes the buttons, and windows glide silently up and down.

The lone woman working at Clark Medical Supply gives her undivided professional attention to each customer, one at a time, unless the telephone rings, at which point she becomes completely focused on that. I wander around, looking at elevated toilet seats and chairs for the shower, wondering if I should buy them, too, as a purchase I had thought would take ten minutes requires an hour, in part because Dr. Singh has not put a diagnosis on the prescription, and this woman, faded but firm, has to have a diagnosis before she can sell Dan a walker. This means her calling Dr. Singh's office and getting a constant busy signal. I try it on my cell phone and get through, but the doctor is not available.

Twice I go outside to give Dan updates. "Get that urinal," he growls the second time, and I run to fetch it from the trunk. "Too late," he says, furious; he has wet his pants.

Finally, the issue becomes clear: if I want Dan's insurance to pay for this item, I have to have a diagnosis. I take out my wallet, find the credit card he and I share, and pay for the walker.

Then the woman has to explain the thing to me and show me how to use it. She carefully installs the wheels on its front legs and packs the non-wheeled attachments into a box.

"My husband is ill," I say for the second time. " We have to go home."

But there are forms to explain and a paper to sign on which I affirm that I have been given all this information. Only then can I put the box in the trunk of the car and drive home.

There I open the walker for Dan, and he ignores it. He falls against the piano bench, cutting his forehead. He starts to feed the dogs and with a twitch of his arm scatters dry dog food across the kitchen floor. Trying to make a tuna salad with the new packaged tuna, he knocks his favorite white mixing bowl onto the floor; it splinters into a dozen pieces.

The dogs are happy to eat off the floor, and the bowl can be replaced. Dan's annoyed because we don't have any scallions for the salad, but he's been annoyed with me for months. What's new is our complete loss of balance, this riptide that's dragging us out to a sea of confusion and disaster. Dan thinks he's returned home to take up life as he left it; I can no longer count on his greater wisdom and common sense. We all, the dogs too, have fallen against the piano bench to be swept away, our feet in the air, our heads on the floor.

Later I bring the pillows from the guestroom into our bedroom so that he can prop himself up farther. He helps me place them. When he lies back, he looks at me.

"Will you take care of me?" he asks in his new voice, no longer slurred so much as broken.

I sit down alongside him, take his hand. "Yes, I'll take care of you." I've loved him for so long; I can't imagine anything else.

The next morning, Thursday, Dan steers the walker out the front door, off the porch, and down the driveway about 20 yards, to the box where the *Times Union* is delivered. He takes the paper out of the box; I move away from the window so he won't see me watching him on his return trip.

In the afternoon we go for a drive, and on our way home, we stop and see Dave, the VW technician who services our two Volkswagens. His shop is in the barn in back of his house. Dan and Dave are on the town Zoning Board of Appeals. Dan chairs the board, and last night was the first ZBA meeting he has ever missed, in about five years; Dave chaired it for him. They are both utterly fascinated by zoning issues, and Dave goes over what happened at the meeting—the board is dealing with two separate applications for gravel mines, always a hot issue, along with the usual setback alterations. I turn off the car, bored by zoning but happy to sit in the shade of Dave's tree-lined driveway while Dan talks to his friend.

Weeks later I tell Dave, "That was our best day," and he says, "Oh, Debby."

Our best, but not a good day. We keep the plastic urinal on Dan's bedside table, but he can't use it if he's asleep, and he never makes it through the night. Beginning on Thursday I strip the bed down to the mattress every morning and launder it all. Friday I add a rubber pad to his side of the bed, hoping he won't notice.

At nine o'clock I call my office and ask for another day off. Dr. Singh has said that a Dr. Toegel will call us. At 9:30 I realize that losing another half day would be foolish, so I call Dr. Toegel, and learn that he has taken the day off and referred Dan's case to his associate Dr. Ehrlich. Both Dr. Ehrlich and his assistant are "in clinic," and no one else can help me, so I do as bidden and leave a message on the assistant's voicemail.

Then Dan asks if I will get the mail and the *Times*, and "while you're out, will you get me some Depends?"

"—Sure." Half an hour later I'm in CVS, studying packages of this product I've never given a thought to. Since Dan is 6 feet tall, I reach for "Large," only to find that these are meant for people who weigh twice what he does. In Depends, Dan is a "Small."

After lunch I call the doctor, get the voicemail, and use the menu to go back to the receptionist; "I have to talk to someone today," I say, trying for a tone that's friendly but urgent. "If Dr. Ehrlich isn't available, I need to speak with someone else."

"She'll call you," snaps the receptionist.

"Give me the voicemail again," I say, without adding *please*, and I leave another message. At three I call again and reach Dr, Ehrlich's assistant. It's not clear from our conversation whether she would have called me, that day or ever, but she does give Dan an appointment for 11:30 the next morning.

I'm relieved but exhausted with this last set of hurdles. Dan wants to have dinner at the Red Barn, and I think, why not. Why not pretend, for a minute here and there, that we're on vacation, that we've taken some time off together to relax and enjoy our house, and we have enough money to eat dinner out every night. He changes his shirt and puts on his spring newsboy cap, of oatmeal Irish linen. I'm adept by now at popping the walker into the back seat when we leave home, then hopping out when we arrive and trotting around the car to snap it open and present it to him as he disembarks. Otherwise he will try to walk without it.

We drive north through a fresh spring evening, and at the Red Barn we get a table by the window. At six o'clock the light outside is as crisp as the air.

"They need to get going on these window boxes," I say, and Dan nods, more interested in the menu. He's keeping his calendar again, morning and evening; he wrote down what we ate that night, but the entries are illegible.

After Dan goes to bed I sit on the couch and read his file from Kingston Hospital. The neurosurgeon reports that in the middle of his examination, Dan turned away and began to eat some food left on his tray and watch television. This night, my life is such that I am relieved to read that: *someone else noticed.*

Dr. Ehrlich's assistant has given us detailed directions to their office building, part of the Albany Medical Center complex. Eleven stoplights down Madison Avenue, she says, and we count them as we go. We get twelve.

Throughout this trip Dan tries to call Paul, who has said that he'll leave his office early and drive up from New York for the afternoon to help us out around the house, then have dinner with us. Now Dan is compelled to try to exchange grid coordinates hourly with Paul.

On an upper floor of an office building, the waiting room is huge and nerve-rackingly full of people. It's finally dawned on me that this is the Friday of a holiday weekend. We've been lucky to get this appointment, safely between Albany's notorious rush hour and the weekend exodus. There is the usual fistful of forms to fill out, which Dan turns over to me. Fine; I can check "yes" for depression.

Dr. Ehrlich is in his mid-thirties, handsome in a slightly soft, Teutonic way. He wears a well-cut suit in a beautiful dark fabric, the kind of suit Dan used to wear when we worked in New York, and the fashionable eyeglasses—with narrow, dark frames—seen in magazine ads.

He examines Dan in much the same way that Dr. Singh did, testing how his eyes track a pen, hammering at his knee. He asks Dan about his symptoms, questions that don't seem probing or detailed, and Dan answers briefly.

Dr. Ehrlich says that he can't make a diagnosis based on the MRI film; he needs to do a brain biopsy. He explains the procedure, one I've never heard of, and its risks; the importance of getting enough of the brain to study, but not too much.

Think about it, he says. But if you decide to go ahead, I wouldn't put it off—I'd have it done in the next week or two.

I should have spoken up. I should have said, but this is a man who skittered up and down the pyramids at Chichen Itza, who shovels snow off our roof in winter, who could recite the twenty-six words of James Coburn's dialogue in *The Magnificent Seven*. Three weeks ago he was running and doing the *Times* crossword puzzle daily. Today he is crippled and no one knows why.

I pushed so hard to get him here, and now I blink. I should have demanded that Dr. Ehrlich admit Dan to the hospital and do the brain biopsy first thing in the morning. But I knew he wouldn't. There was protocol to think of and a holiday weekend and Dan wanting to get home for Paul and nobody ready to face this today except, possibly, me. Dr. Ehrlich says he will speak to Dr. Singh on Tuesday. We start back home, Dan wildly calling Paul on the cell phone and then telling me to stop at the liquor store so we'll have plenty of gin. At the shopping center he waves away the walker. "I'll use you!"

So we stagger along like something out of Beckett, across the parking lot and into the store, a quarter-acre of glass bottles.

"Hurt your leg?" says Bill, who's on the counter today.

"Don't-know, what's-wrong," says Dan. "Been-to-the-doctor."

"I hope they find out soon," says Bill, his whole face narrow with concern.

"That stare," Bill says to me much later. I nod and turn away, so that he won't say the rest. *Like a trapped animal.*

At home I call Dr. Singh's office and learn that they have not received the final pathology report—the one that might confirm MS—so it will be Tuesday before that comes in. Paul's been delayed in leaving the city, so he drives up through the evening's heaviest traffic, arriving not at three but at seven. He keeps in touch by cell phone, and Dan pesters me every 15 minutes to call the Red Barn and tell them we're still coming. I do call once, afraid we'll be shut out on the holiday weekend, but we aren't, and dinner goes well enough. Paul and Dan have known each other for 30 years, since they first worked together at McGraw Hill. Now Paul is editor in chief at a smaller press and recently hired Dan to ghostwrite the section on "water" for a book titled *Chemical and Biological Warfare: A Comprehensive Survey for the Concerned Citizen*. When Dan goes to New York weekends to work for *Time* he stays in Brooklyn with Paul and his wife, Denise, and their son, Ben, who is almost three.

"You're probably horrified," I say, while Dan is in the restroom after dinner.

"—Not horrified," Paul says carefully. "But I think you should come to New York, to Memorial Sloan-Kettering. You could stay with us for as long as you want. You and the dogs."

I try to visualize this exceedingly generous, impractical offer.

"Did you ever meet my friend Giselle?" Paul is saying. "No, she joined the book club after you and Dan moved out of the city. She works in communications at MSK. I'll call her tomorrow."

Back home, Dan doesn't use the walker, and he falls. Paul is a couple of inches taller than he and outweighs him by 50 pounds, so he can lift him under the arms and sit him on the couch. "You have to use the walker, Dan," he snaps. "*Use the walker.*"

Then Paul leaves, to go home to his family and their holiday weekend. I stand in the driveway, watching the red taillights disappear up the hill. I swallow hard and tell myself we are not abandoned in the outback, we have plenty of friends here, and Paul has promised to be back Monday afternoon to mow the lawn. "Make a list of chores you want me to do," he said.

I do keep a list that weekend, in pencil on a piece of scrap paper, but it's titled "symptoms worse," so that when I talk to the doctors on Tuesday I will be a well-organized caregiver and not forget anything. It goes like this:

—speech difficult, hard to understand

—fingers don't work—uses utensils awkwardly, needs help getting dressed

—eats with difficulty, chewing, swallowing—coughs as eats

—eats sloppily—food goes onto table, floor/drools

—uses walker w/ difficulty—balance v. poor

—I can't take him anywhere by myself—his balance too poor, I can't manage him

—falls frequently in house

—depressed

—incontinence—tries not to, but pees in bed every night

—toilet stops up often—uses more toilet paper than he realizes?

—grabbed towel rack for balance, pulled it out of wall; looked at me, frightened, tragic at the loss, when he couldn't force it back up

—knocked bottled water from shelf, it cracked, leaking 2 gallons onto floor near electric heater

I don't write down those last three things, but they happen too.

Saturday's mail brings some work for him, the last few pages of a book that he's to check. He smiles at it weakly, as if it's an old friend he can no longer help.

Today is also an anniversary for us, of sorts. Twenty-four years ago, Dan moved into my apartment in New York. I had no money then, as I never have, so my welcome presents for him were a poem, an ink pad, and a rubber stamp with his new address. Since the holiday is a floating one, so is our anniversary, and we never paid much attention to it.

We never paid much attention to marriage either. Dan had been married before, so he felt that he had had that experience, and I had no interest in it. We didn't want to have children, so I saw no reason to make the relationship official. Twice over the years we considered marrying for the health insurance, but when I was young and freelancing I found the idea distasteful, and later, when I was salaried and he wasn't, there was no saving in his going on my policy, so the moment passed again. Eighteen years ago when we bought this house as a second home, I made a will, leaving Dan my minuscule estate and pointing out to him this administrative kindness. "If you don't write a will," I said, "everything you have will go to your mother." He looked appropriately horrified, but he never did anything about it. Since we held the house, our major asset, jointly, I didn't press him.

Sunday I go to church. I pray for strength and courage for both of us. To pray, *please let Dan get well,* already seems preposterous, like praying for peace while I duck carpet-bombing. Better to pray for something that I need that I might get.

My mother calls, to see what we're doing on our holiday weekend, and I figure I'd better tell her that Dan is sick.

"I knew it," she says. "I knew something was wrong with him on Mother's Day. Remember, I called you later, and I said—"

"Yes, I remember."

We hang up; she calls back ten minutes later.

"Can you do Dan's work for him? So they'll keep paying him?"

"No. No, I can't do that." *We're not that desperate.*

Margaret calls. Their friends Ken and Carol are visiting from Rhode Island for the weekend. They'll all come over tonight with a pork roast, she says, "cooked, ready to serve. We'll bring the vegetables, salad, paper plates. You won't have to do a thing."

"You told Ken and Carol that Dan is sick?"

"Yeah. They're cool."

Ken and Carol are cool, which is to say they are warm, engaging and friendly and pleased to be in the country. As Margaret and Steven are dark-haired and short—Steven my height, Margaret tiny—so Carol and Ken are tall and fair, in the way of people who have never lived in New York City. Carol sits next to Dan at the table and does an artful job of including him in the conversation without requiring him to talk much. The only bad time is when Dan suddenly lurches across the kitchen with Steven's martini glass in his hand. I'm standing at the counter and see him coming toward me, straining at the effort—

"Dan—not with a glass in your hand!" I hate the desperation in my voice, our humiliation as talk at the table stops, but all I can see is blood.

"Let me make you another one, Dan," says Steven, getting up. "I'll fix them both."

After dinner, Dan retires to the bedroom and the NCAA finals without saying good night. The rest of us sit around the table. I make coffee and find the paper cups left over from last summer's picnics at Jacob's Pillow.

"He's still a good host," says Margaret. "He wanted to keep our glasses full."

"He had me take the cheese out early," I say. "I wouldn't have remembered."

Paul arrives Monday afternoon, and the three of us move in and around the house like people under water. Visiting Dan that summer was a series of snapshots from hell, Paul says later. "But in those 48 hours . . ." He shakes his head. *That was the worst.*

Paul mows the lawns while Dan sits on the deck. "Plenty of gas in this, Dan," says Paul, as if reassuring him that when he wants to use it next week, it will be ready. I put tomato plants into the raised beds outside the fence.

Dan goes back indoors, lies down in front of the television. Paul and I work out front. He rakes up the longest grass; I use it as mulch on the tomatoes.

"If you get a chance," I say, "will you speak to Dan about a Health Care Proxy?"

"Doesn't have one? . . . Why do I even ask."

Paul is out back by the compost bins, rescuing the pitchfork. Dan put it in the middle of the fenced bin one day this spring, where I can neither reach nor use it.

"He wants to go to Gigi's for dinner," I say, wondering if Paul can face this. "It's on your way home."

"Fine," says Paul, "let's."

But Gigi's is closed for the holiday and so is everything else. I walk in and out of the house, calling restaurants, feeling solely responsible for putting together some mutually acceptable dinner plans, until I find the Beekman, our decent, if unexciting fallback.

Paul sits in the living room looking at the *Times* while I walk the dogs. As we come back down the hill I can hear the strains of Gavin Bryars's "Jesus' Blood Never Failed Me Yet." This seems perfectly normal to me—for months, Dan has been listening to everything at ear-splitting volume, and he and I both found this CD bizarre but compelling—but it doesn't to Paul.

"I thought he had gone completely around the bend," he says later. "He had this odd little smile on his face, and he put on this lunatic music—"

Typically, Dan did not say to Paul, Let me play you this weird CD that Deb and I heard on the radio one Sunday as we were driving home from Vermont. We liked it so much that I went online the next day and bought it. Typically, Dan just put the CD on for Paul without introduction—the way, come to think of it, that Dan and I first heard the piece on the radio, tuning in on it midway, to a British tramp not quite singing, not quite saying,

Jesus' Blood never failed me yet
Never failed me yet
Jesus' blood never failed me yet
There's one thing I know
For he loves me so . . .

to string accompaniment or a cappella, in a repeated loop that runs for more than an hour. Tom Waits is dubbed in with the tramp toward the end and then sings the final part by himself.

Dan is still a good host. He remembers that he and Paul share a love of music, all kinds, that in their years in New York they might stand in joints for hours to hear this bassist, that pianist. He is a friend, if a sometimes manipulative one. He wants to show Paul the music.

At the Beekman we're given a table in the back by the bar. Always before we've sat out front, where the light pours in on a dining solarium, but today this room is quiet, a peaceful den. Dan orders a steak and works at cutting it.

Paul tries. "You know, Dan, you'll probably have to go back into the hospital. Even if just for this test, this—brain biopsy. And if you do, you should have a Health Care Proxy. It just lets them know what you want them to do. Otherwise, you're letting them make the decisions."

Dan nods, his only reaction. I have no idea what his paranoia index might be, but I can imagine one, can imagine his thinking of Paul and me as coconspirators. The talk moves on—Paul's work, mutual friends. Paul and I finish our meals before Dan does, and I hate to think of him struggling to keep up.

"You could take that home," I said, touching his elbow, "eat it later, or tomorrow. There's no need to rush."

Immediately he starts to take big pieces of meat and stuff them into his mouth, chewing ferociously, staring intently at me.

"I'm not in any hurry, Dan," says Paul, who faces a 90-mile drive through holiday traffic. "Slow down."

Dan would have continued to chew big chunks of beef except that he coughs, spraying sauce onto the plate in front of him.

We get through coffee, the bill. Paul escorts us to the car, folds up the walker. "Call me," he says. "I feel like you're besieged with calls. I'll keep after Giselle," his friend at MSK, "and you call me."

As we drive out of Rhinebeck, Dan says, "Twenty minutes earlier and we could have seen *Enigma*," which is showing at the theater here, where we saw *Nine Queens* four weeks ago.

"That's all right," I say. "Better to spend the time with Paul." I'm thinking, what is he thinking? How I would get him in and out of the theater? He would have fallen asleep anyway.

What he's thinking is the way life used to be. When he was sharp, when he tracked things, when he would herd Paul and me, who counted on his encyclopedic knowledge and interests, to this concert or that movie.

Hardly do we have this exchange when he dozes off. Without the dogs, we can have the windows down, and the sweet May air fills the car. The clouds are blushed with the sunset. I turn off the radio. Dan sleeps beside me. I drive, holding onto these minutes.

Paul's right about the swell of calls, which grows to a flood in the next week. Anita, too, thinks we should go to Memorial Sloan-Kettering. Margaret reports that AARP has designated NYU Medical Center as one of the top ten hospitals in the country. Josh says he knows just the doctor we need in New York; he'll call him and get back to us.

I thank them. I imagine pulling up in front of MSK or NYU in my red Jetta. Then what? Dan staggers in on his walker while I look for a parking place?

It wouldn't be like that. Paul would help. Margaret would help.

Georgia, my boss, sees only doctors in New York—the "real doctors," she calls them. But Georgia has a flexible schedule and plenty of money. By moving up here permanently nine years ago, Dan and I burned our medical bridges. This is where we live now. This is where we work, where we shop, and where we go to the doctor.

Missing among the calls is Dan's mother. I don't know what to tell her, so I don't tell her anything.

I have told my father, a retired physician, long divorced from my mother, and he and my stepmother call every evening for an update. Despite hearing aids in both ears, telephone calls are difficult for him. I elevate my voice. He listens hard. He refers to Dr. Singh as "this gal in Kingston." I wince. He asks cogent questions and listens to my answers. He is horrified that Dan has been released from Kingston Hospital, and he is furious about the walker and the physical therapy. "That's not treatment!" he says. "He needs treatment!" This is a new role for him, at 87; always before, he has defended the practice of medicine.

He tells Maria, my half sister, and she calls Monday evening, after we return from the Beekman. She and her husband, Jon, are scheduled to fly to Colorado on Wednesday for a week's vacation.

"Do you think we shouldn't go?" she asks.

"Of course you should go," I say, wishing desperately that she would stay.

"I'm off work starting tomorrow," she says. "I could come down and see you."

"Maria's coming tomorrow," I tell Dan, knowing this will cheer him. Maria is 33, and he loves her like a daughter. Anyone would. She's a park ranger, first for Boulder City Parks, now administrating a dozen state parks in Vermont. Managing thousands of acres and the millions of people who visit them has made her cheerful, calm, well-organized, good humored, able to focus the moment but never lose sight of the big picture.

Tuesday morning I call Dr. Singh's office. She's not in today, the receptionist tells me confidently, but I reach the doctor with the beeper number she gave me the day we first went to Kingston; it sounds as if she's in a car.

"I'll have my office call you today as soon as the test result comes."

"His symptoms get worse every day."

"Like what."

I read to her from my list. At "coughs when he eats" she says, "Give him puréed food."

Puréed food?

"If you can't do that, feed him baby food."

At "falls in the house" she says, "Do you want a wheelchair?"

"No, I don't want a wheelchair, I want a diagnosis and treatment." I take a breath. "My father, who is a retired physician, thinks I should take Dan to Albany Medical Center." I hate giving a no-confidence vote in the middle of a crisis, but it's been three days, for God's sake, I had to talk to someone.

"The trouble with that is they'll do everything all over again, all the tests," she says. "I will speak to Dr. Ehrlich."

I don't care if they do all the tests again, but I know what she means. They would do a third MRI and say they couldn't diagnose him without a brain biopsy. They would test him for Lyme again, and again find that he doesn't have it. The point is not a third round of the same tests, but to go forward from what's been done.

"Did you call the physical therapist?" she asks.

"I don't know any physical therapists in this area."

"Call the hospital! Make an appointment there. It's very important that he start physical therapy."

Georgia calls from the office. She's back from a vacation, and Elliot must have updated her. She's concerned: "What can we do for you?"

"—Give me a couple more days."

Maria arrives from her home in the southern Adirondacks, two hours north of us. She embraces Dan, who's sitting in the wooden rocker on the deck, and admires the new perennials, still in their pots. "They're fine," she says. We make sandwiches and bring them outdoors. The day is cloudy but mild, finally a harbinger of summer.

The laundry finishes and I bring the basket of wet clothes up from the cellar. "Dryer isn't working again," I say. "Heats up but doesn't rotate. I'll call—Dan!"

He's staggering toward the cellar stairs.

"Don't go down there!" I plead. The cellar entry was originally outdoors. We had the screened porch built over it with lift-up doors above the stairway—Dan's design. But the steps are still rough, uneven stones. Maria doesn't say a word, just follows behind Dan, gently grasping the waistband of his pants as they take the steps one at a time.

They're sitting on the deck again when I come back from hanging laundry.

"Am I right?"

He nods.

When Dan gets up, without a word, and starts inside, Maria and I follow him. He's fallen against the walker, and now the left side of it won't extend to the correct angle, turning it into more of a danger than an assist. Dan lies down in the bedroom. Maria and I sit at the kitchen table; she keeps her voice level.

"I think what I should do," she says, "is stop by and see Dad on my way home."

Grateful, I copy my list for her. We kiss good-bye. "My bet is, Dad will come down and see you," she says, partly as a warning.

An hour later my father calls. Maria's standing next to him, and it sounds as if he's still reading the list as he talks.

"He has to go to the hospital! This is not a case for home care."

"The brain biopsy is the next step. Dr. Singh said she'd set that up with Dr. Ehrlich—"

"This gal in Kingston."

"—Yes. She doesn't want Dan to have the biopsy in Kingston. I'll call her again now. If she doesn't come through, we'll go to Albany."

I reach Dr. Singh through her beeper. She hasn't been able to make contact with Dr. Ehrlich. She will call him again tomorrow.

I know we can't continue like this. With the words "puréed food," Dr. Singh cast us out on a riptide as firmly as Dr. Hahn did by handing out Pletal. But just in case I'm wrong, praying that I'm wrong, I call Susan and Ed, our medical friends. "I need to find a physical therapist—can you recommend anyone?"

"I really don't know anybody," Susan says, "but Ed will. Let me get him."

"Nah, I don't know anybody in particular," says Ed. He sounds tired. "Just call the hospital, they're good there."

I hang up, my face crumpling into a sob. I'm sitting on the couch in the living room. Dan and the dogs are stretched out on the bed, watching the NCAA finals. I have to get used to this. People are not at my beck and call. This is my problem, not theirs.

At night, Dan still sleeps on his left side, knees bent. I curl next to him, my right arm around his waist. He holds my right hand in his; we lace our fingers. Cooper sleeps on the other side of Dan, the first line of defense between his pack and the door. Lulu settles with a sigh between our legs. The house is black these cloudy nights, the temperature in the low 60s, warm enough to leave the doors and windows open to the screens. Peepers cry from the pond across the road. A tear slides from under my eyelid.

I keep Dan's calendar now—he never touches it. On Wednesday, the bills for our two telephone lines are due, along with his health insurance premium. I ask him to pay them, feeling like Simon Legree—if Dan isn't working, he isn't making any money—but he has $12,000 in his checking account and I have $100 in mine, until I get paid on Friday. He writes the checks slowly, trying hard, but his handwriting is so messy that Verizon gives him a $2 credit the next month.

I call the hospital in Hudson. The absurdity of making an appointment for physical therapy for a person who loses mobility daily from a problem that no one can identify is enough to make me lightheaded, but never let it be said I was uncooperative about Dan's care.

Which again is out of my hands. The physical therapy department has an opening in mid-June, but they need a diagnosis.

"He doesn't have a diagnosis yet."

"It should be right there on your prescription."

"It's not," I say, looking at the prescription in my hand.

"We can't treat him without it."

"We'll have it by the time he gets there."

I'm making our lunch, tears rolling down my cheeks. No doctor has called, and more important, neither has my father. I had been so sure that he would, to tell me he was on his way down, ready to offer parental support and doctorly advice. But he and my stepmother are visiting a friend whose husband is in the hospital. They're helping her with shopping and housework. Then they'll take care of Maria and Jon's dog while they're away. They have their own concerns.

Determined not to be overwhelmed, I decide, with Margaret's telephonic encouragement, to try to exchange

Dan's walker for an undented one. True, he caused the damage, but "they'll exchange it," says Margaret. "They don't want him to fall."

By now I'm nervous about leaving Dan alone. I call Rob; he and his wife, Anita, have been friends for years. They drew us up here and live only a couple of miles away. I kiss Dan good-bye. "Rob will stop by soon." The dogs watch me, their brows furrowed, from their stations on the bed—Cooper alongside Dan, Lulu on top of his legs.

I drive to Clark Medical Supply, and just as I do every minute—driving, walking the dogs, folding the laundry—any time I'm not actively talking to someone—I ask myself if I should be doing something else. Should I take Dan to New York? Josh hasn't called back with a doctor. Paul's friend Giselle no longer works for MSK. Should I take Dan to Boston? He'd be close there to his family in Worcester. To NYU? Should I be driving him to Albany this minute? Dad's right, Dan should be in the hospital . . . wouldn't Dr. Singh and Dr. Ehrlich put him in the hospital? What if they didn't? What if they said, He's not sick enough to be in the hospital? Should I take him to New York? Boston?

At Clark nothing has changed. After 15 minutes—one customer, two telephone calls—it's my turn.

The clerk, still a shadow of a woman, but a firm shadow, frowns at the walker. "He fell on it?"

"—Yes." Damn, I should have lied.

She shakes her head—"I can't just give him a new one"—and calls the owner of the store for a consult. He directs her to call the doctor and get a new prescription. Dr. Singh is in her office and won't give Dan a prescription for another walker. "Not if he's falling on it," she says to me when I take the phone. "He has to have a wheelchair."

I give the phone back to the clerk. "I don't want a wheelchair today," I say, thinking of our small house, its carpeted floors, and of Dan, who needs to be in a hospital, not a wheelchair. "I'll just take this back." I avert my face, folding up the walker. I will not cry in front of her.

"I can't let you do that," she says. "I can't let you take damaged goods."

It must be adrenaline that makes me think fast. "We bought this," I say, "remember? We didn't have a diagnosis, so we had to pay for it. It's mine. I'm taking it home."

Her look grieves for me. She must see desperate people all the time.

Approaching our house, I can feel my heart lift at the sight of two extra vehicles in the driveway: Rob's pickup truck and my father's Saab. They've come!

Inside, no one smiles back at me. My father and stepmother meet me in the kitchen. They've grown shorter in their old age, but they haven't diminished. My father has a full head of white hair and a square white beard. Today he's in tears.

Rob is sitting in the bedroom easy chair with a book, facing Dan, looking grim. I lean over the bed to kiss Dan. The dogs don't move.

"No luck," I say, indicating the walker. "Dr. Singh wanted you to have a wheelchair."

Dan gives me a look like, *yeah, right.*

Rob leaves then; he's not one to chat, but I fear disapproval. My parents don't stay long, and later what my father recalls of that afternoon is the dogs. "Those dogs," he says to me several times, "those dogs knew something was wrong with him." Probably the dogs didn't leave the bed, even when they heard someone come in the back door. Cooper may have growled, a mean rumble deep in his throat, and Dan grasped his collar. Probably when the old people turned the corner into the bedroom, the first thing they saw was three silent beings on watch, without a welcoming look among them. Probably a moment passed before Dan croaked hello.

Now we're alone again, and I sit on the edge of the bed, facing him. "My father's very worried about you," I say.

Dan nods. In their own reserved way, he and my father like each other.

"I know I said I would take care of you." My voice breaks and the tears start. "But I think taking care of you now means taking you to the hospital."

He nods. "Tomorrow," he says.

"I think he wanted to finish the pork you left us and watch the NCAA finals," I say to Margaret on the phone that evening.

"Good for him."

It's eight o'clock and I'm sitting at the kitchen table, Dan's desk calendar fanned before me.

I'd been reheating Margaret's pork and squash in the oven when I saw him stagger, without his walker, through the living room on his way to the bathroom. I followed him, gently clasping the waistband of his pants. He stopped at the desk and started to turn the pages of his calendar, which was held to its plastic base by only one metal clasp. As he stabbed at the pages with his fingers, the clasp came loose and the calendar pages scattered on the desk. In trying to get them together again, he made things worse; the pages kept slipping from his fingers. I picked up the ones that fell onto the floor, and as he tried to interleave them again they became only more disordered. A urine stain was spreading on his pants, and he would not leave the calendar.

"Sweetie, go pee, you can fix this later."

He didn't acknowledge me, just kept moving the calendar pages around.

Eventually, he peed and changed his pants and came to the dinner table with the calendar scooped in both hands. I had cut up his meat so he wouldn't have to struggle with it, and he kept working on the calendar as he ate, wrinkling the pages, spotting some with pork gravy. From my seat I could see where he was going wrong, but there was no doing it for him. I ate my dinner in the silence. I made coffee; we finished the last of a blueberry pie. With his final bite, he abandoned the calendar and went to bed.

Now I play a sort of chronological solitaire as I call Margaret, Paul, Anita, and Linda. I stack the pages by month on the kitchen table. I answer my friends' sensible questions, am sustained by their concern. I start to put the days in order. By nine o' clock my friends have given me the strength to call my mother.

"Get those . . . what are they, they're not doctors but they're not nurses either, they come with the ambulance," she says.

"EMTs."

"What?"

"Emergency medical technicians."

"That's right. They were so wonderful when John fell. They took him to the hospital. I don't know what I would have done. I couldn't pick him up—"

She continues with the story of my stepfather's dreadful 2 a.m. fall the previous summer and the intelligence and kindness of the EMTs, a story that takes place in real time and one I've heard before, but I'm thinking, she has a point. If the local rescue squad transports Dan to Albany Medical Center, he's more likely to get attention.

". . . good idea . . ." July and August are still completely missing from the calendar. "I'll speak with Dan about it in the morning." I crawl under his big wooden desk to look for them.

"But what if he doesn't want to?"

The pages have slipped off the back of the desk, onto the sliver of floor between it and the wall. "Then I'll drive him."

"Oh, I hate to think of your doing that. The parking there is just awful."

"It's 9:30. I'll deal with it in the morning."

I'm too drained now to call anyone else, but I have found every single day of the calendar and put them in order. I double-check them as I leave a message for Elliott at the office. Then I struggle to put the pages back on the plastic base. Part of the problem is its age; he should have a new one. Finally, I have it back on his desk, just as it's always been.

"Ma had a good idea," I say the next morning at breakfast. "We can get you a rescue squad transport."

Dan shakes his head.

"They'll bring you right in. You won't have to wait."

He shakes his head, eyes on his English muffin.

"—OK . . . Are you scared?"

"Nope," he says with another little shake of his head.

I'm suffused with apprehension (what if they don't admit him? what if they do?), but I don't pursue the topic. A few months ago I bought a book titled *Be Not Afraid: Overcoming the Fear of Death*.

"Are you afraid of dying?" he asked.

"Yes," I said, surprised at his surprise.

He said nothing more, and I assumed he had found yet another flaw in me.

While Dan is showering, my mother calls. "Are you going to use the rescue squad?"

"No, he doesn't want to."

"Oh, I wish he would. You'll have to park across the street—"

"Ma, he's agreed to go to the hospital. I'm not going to argue with him about how he gets there."

In the bathroom Dan's spraying his beard and what's left of his hair with the witch hazel spray he likes—not lightly, as usual, but carefully and repeatedly.

He smiles back at me with a shrug. "Might have to last for a while."

I take the dogs for a final walk, and as we come back in the door, the phone rings; it's Georgia, at the office.

"Elliot will take you to New York," she says. "He'll drive you down today."

"—That's very kind, Georgia. But we're going to Albany. We're about to leave."

"Then take down the names of these doctors I found."

She begins reading me names and telephone numbers. As I write, I realize these are names my officemate Mike already e-mailed me—he got them off a Web site—but there's no stopping Georgia. While I'm on the phone, Dan takes off Lulu's leash, which means I then have to chase her around the house. She runs like a maniac, knowing it's Crate Time. I finally catch her by closing the bedroom door on us. I stand for a moment, holding her in my arms, my cheek against the smooth triangle of her head, before

I open the door.

"Call-Dr.-Singh?" says Dan. After twenty-five days of this dreadful illness, he can still pose a question that is meant as an order.

"No," I say. "We don't owe her anything."

And we set off. At the post office, I smile to myself. Of course he didn't want to ride up with the rescue squad; they wouldn't have stopped for the mail and the *Times*.

Albany, June

Today, we don't count the stoplights.

The entrance to the emergency room is lined with signs suggesting that if I leave the car there for more than ten seconds it will be firebombed from an upper story. I run to the hospital door in search of a wheelchair . . . discharged patients are always wheeled to the door . . . no wheelchair.

So much for my plan. I run back to the car, where Dan is disembarking. I give him the walker and walk alongside him toward the entry, a large revolving door flanked by doors that open inward with the push of a button. A black man in green scrubs, talking on a cell phone, pushes the button for us.

"This is an emergency admission," I say to him. "We need help."

He clicks off the phone and guides Dan through the doors. I run back to the car. A small parking area at the end of the drive is full. I drive out, across the street to a multistoried parking garage. I take the suitcase out of the trunk, then go to the passenger side to put the newspaper and two envelopes of MRI film into a tote bag. With my head in the car, I hear a horrible crunch.

"Stop!" I shriek.

Too late; a young woman in a red SUV has backed out of a parking slot at a right angle to me and rolled into the suitcase. "Sorry!" she says, and drives off.

The *Follies* case, the Callas case, *O Brother Where Art Thou*, all cracked. Nothing to do about it now; layered with the suitcase, tote bag, pocketbook, I run down the ramp, cross the street on a red light, and trot back into the hospital.

Inside, I follow red arrows until I arrive at a small waiting room with a stretch of glass-walled office on one side. Dan is sitting inside this office. I wave to him. He leans forward to open the door for me and falls on the floor.

A male aide buzzes me in and helps Dan back into the chair. A woman materializes with a clipboard. Dan's his own rescue squad: *Let's move these two along.*

The woman shows us to a white-sheeted gurney in a hallway. We sit on it side by side, our legs dangling. I make us a little camp, with the newspapers next to us, the walker leaning against the wall.

Men and women wearing white outfits or green scrubs pass in front of us, back and forth on their brisk official way. The nurses here don't wear caps, they wear white pants and smocks that are often patterned with teddy bears or flowers. Almost immediately a group is shown to the gurney next to ours. An elderly man in a wheelchair is accompanied by two women, one of them also older, evidently his wife, the other much younger. The older couple have full heads of hair, pure white, and narrow, fine faces with high cheekbones and ivory skin. They've dressed for this occasion as if for lunch at a country club forty years ago, in navy blue blazers, he with gray slacks, a pale blue shirt, and a striped tie; she with a navy blue A-line skirt and a white blouse with a round collar, stockings and navy blue flats. Her legs are good; years of tennis and golf. She's carrying *The New Yorker*, and she stands next to the man and looks at it with him, page by page, reading him the captions on the cartoons. The younger woman, in brown slacks and a brown checked blouse that can only be called ugly, sits on the bed, turning pages in a three-ring binder.

Dan has discovered, on the wall next to us, three boxes of purple disposable gloves. Ever since we waited for Dr. Singh in the examining room in Kingston Hospital, I've been fascinated by those gloves. They look nothing so much as edible, succulently delicious, like some new sorbet, and I'm not surprised when Dan starts with the smallest size, removing two gloves from the box and silently pulling them onto his hands. It takes a bit of tugging; I help him, pushing gently the notch between each finger. He spreads his fingers in front of him, then turns his hands over. We gaze at the purple rubber stretched tight over his palms. He takes the gloves off, pulling at each finger carefully, and gives them to me. Since they're no longer sanitary, and there's no trash basket in sight, I put them in my bag. We can use them at home.

Next he takes two medium-sized gloves out of the box and pulls them on. I'm aware of the group next to us watching this, but I don't care. It's all I can do not to nibble his fingertips, to see if the gloves are grape, or plum.

The medium gloves fit better, reaching to his wrists . . . a nurse interviews the group at the next bed . . . Dan peels off the gloves . . . the younger woman is a private-duty nurse . . . I put the gloves into my bag . . . the man has suffered diarrhea this morning . . . the biggest gloves fit best, Dan has no trouble pulling them on . . . the man's doctor told them to come to the emergency room . . . we admire the perfect fit of the gloves on Dan's long fingers, slender and straight . . .

A Dr. Matthew Damon is introducing himself to us. Young, brown hair, pleasantly square face.

"You like those gloves, Mr. Zinkus?"

Dan is silent, admiring the gloves.

"They're so beautiful," I say hastily. "We can't resist them."

Dr. Damon smiles. "I'm going to ask you to take the gloves off now, Mr. Zinkus, as it were, so I can see your hands. You can keep them." He peels the gloves off as he speaks and lays them neatly at Dan's side. Dan gives them to me; I put them in my bag.

Dr. Damon asks Dan to track his pen without moving his head . . . the nurse leaves the group next to us and the older woman hikes herself up onto the gurney, alongside the private-duty nurse . . . I answer the questions . . . the women next to us are silent, as I was when they spoke . . . I tell the story of the May 6 run. I read my list of worsening symptoms . . . Dr. Damon listens. He takes some notes.

"Anything else?" he says.

" —Sometimes . . . there's a certain, sudden, obsessive attention to something . . . at an inappropriate time and place."

I'm thinking of the calendar, last night, and I'm unable to speak of him in the third person, to say *he has*. Everything else I've told Dr. Damon, Dan knows.

"Boy, I'm glad she said that," says the private duty nurse.

Dr. Damon goes away to look at the MRI film. Dan and I are starving, but I'm afraid to leave him to fetch the lunch from the car. What if they have more questions? What if they take him somewhere and I can't find him? What if we lose our place on whatever routing they have here?

Dr. Damon returns. Yes, the MRI shows an abnormality. "It's interesting," he says to me. He pauses. "That doesn't mean it's good for the patient." To Dan he says, "I've asked for a neurological consult, Mr. Zinkus. Dr. Meredith, the head of neurology, may see you." He turns back to me. "We'll admit him."

Thank God. Admit him. Interesting. Head of neurology.

Dan doesn't see the head of neurology, that day, or ever, as far as I know. He is examined by two neurologists that Saturday, both of them Russian. One is the resident on duty, a pale woman whose every feature—eyes, mouth, hair—suggests exhaustion, whose accent is parsable. The other is a tall man with a red face, a bald pink scalp and shocks of white hair—thick eyebrows, handlebar moustache, and tufts that stick out over his ears.

"Good afternoon!" he fairly shouts. "Very busy here! They ask me to help! Now you must try to talk to me, even though you cannot understand a word I say!"

He's right. But he is fluent. When I get to "coughs when eats" on my list, he says, "Then we cannot feed him! He is at risk for aspiration pneumonia! I will give order, no solid food!"

So we don't eat the lunch sitting in the cooler in the car, or anything else. I never eat in front of Dan again. Looking back, I would give anything to have skipped the suitcase until later and brought the lunch in right away. We could have sat on the gurney and eaten our sandwiches, the last solid food Dan would have in his life.

But it could have killed him.

Which might not have been the worst thing.

I've never heard of aspiration pneumonia, and I think I must have misunderstood the words, but I haven't.

At some point over Memorial Day weekend, Dan had stopped swallowing correctly; every time he ate or drank, three times a day, he inhaled bits of food and liquid into his lungs. That's what made him cough. That's why Dr. Singh said to feed him puréed food. She knew the risk.

Our neighbors in blue disappear at some point during all this, and eventually Dan's given a tiny private room that's part of the ER. It's just large enough for a bed and three walls of sink and examination equipment. There's no place to set down anything—the suitcase, the MRI film the Russian doctor has insisted we take back—"Valuable! To you! We will lose, you keep!"—and it has no window. Dan stretches out on the bed. An aide brings me a straight chair. I leave the door ajar; otherwise the room is claustrophobic.

"Get the lunch?" Dan croaks.

"You're not supposed to eat anything. I'm sorry."

Dr. Damon comes by. "I'm going off now," he says, "but the doctors on duty know you're here. You'll be moved to a room as soon as possible." He shakes hands with Dan, with me. "Good luck," he says.

"So," growls Dan, "that was Matt Damon." He can't really laugh, but I can, only mildly hysterical, admiring what I missed, what he saw immediately.

At five I kiss him good-bye. Again, I try to hold him; again, all he wants is our cell phone. He said he wasn't scared. I leave the door open.

At home Lulu springs from her crate, and even Cooper, half blind, welcomes me ecstatically. Basenjis' tails curl over their backs, and they wag them with effort, only when they're really, really excited. There are fourteen messages on the answering machine, ten of which are real, from the man who's ready to repair the clothes dryer to Matt and Julie, starting on their trip east, to Jan, Dr. Ehrlich's assistant. She has made Dan an appointment for an outpatient brain biopsy for next Thursday, June 6. On Monday Dan is due at the hospital at 7 a.m. for pretesting. I leave her a message, that Dan has been admitted to AMC.

The other calls are from family and friends, and I begin a long series of nights—weeks of nights—in which I do nothing but talk on the phone. I know I should spread this out, ask friends to call other friends. But most of them I want to talk to myself. Most of them I want in the room with me. The needy get cut to alternate nights—my mother—or weekly—Sonia.

On this night, my mother says, "Why don't you kennel the dogs at their vet. I'll pay for it. That way you can stay at the hospital as long as you want. It's very important, you know, to visit people when they're in the hospital. It means a lot to them."

"Thank you. I'll think about it." Lulu is sitting on my lap, Cooper curled next to me. "We're coming up on a weekend, I can handle them for a while."

Dan's mother, Jane, answers the phone and we chat, but unable to keep up a lie, I ask for Judy, his sister. "Dan's in the hospital," I tell her.

"Oh?" she says, in a tone that combines disbelief with dismissal. "What's up?"

I talk, and Judy listens, silent. The only questions she asks are his room and telephone number, neither of which I have.

"I'm writing everything down," Judy says finally, "so I can tell her."

Jane and Judy live together in Worcester, Massachusetts, where Judy and Dan grew up. Judy retired last year after more than 30 years of teaching elementary school. In contrast, Dan had accepted a full scholarship to Columbia, moved to New York, and never looked back. We see them at Thanksgiving, Christmas, Mother's Day, and once in the summer.

They'll visit him over the weekend, says Judy. What are visiting hours?

The next morning I call Elliot at the office and report on Dan's admission. It's Friday, May 31. "I need one more day."

"—All right," he says, with some reluctance. "I guess a walk would be nice."

A walk. By myself, without the dogs straining on their leads, each one with its own agenda. I don't have time for such an extravagance, but maybe I can plant the ornamental grass and the Cobitti daisy, still in their pots.

Dan calls, his voice a whisper. "I still don't have a room."

He spent all night in the little room. He hasn't had anything to eat.

"I'm on my way."

I shower and dress carefully, in Eileen Fisher pants of lavender blue and a white T-shirt. I'm aware of making a personal appearance in a weird kind of theater; not an audition, we passed that yesterday and now we're on a new stage, one on which I attempt to represent, with every detail, what and who we are. I put on the silver ring with its diamond chip that Dan gave me for my birthday this year, and small fake diamond stud earrings that my mother handed off to me. Dan has given me almost all the jewelry I own, most of it silver, all of it "real." Daily, I wear earrings he's given me—until now, when for weeks I wear these fake diamonds, night and day, with pants and skirts, with jeans and a sweatshirt on a cold, rainy Sunday in June. I wear them to work, to the hospital, to the Social Security office, to the nursing homes I tour. I don't know why I can't take them off until months later when I see an ad in the *Times*:

> When in doubt, wear diamonds.
>
> —*Kept Couture*

At the hospital, Dan has disappeared from the emergency room, assigned to a fifth-floor room in the same wing. When I find him, he's twisted away from the door, trying to grab the telephone, just out of reach on a stand by his bed.

"Where were you?" he croaks.

I tell him how far I walked the dogs. I give him the mail and the newspapers. His nurse, Phyllis, introduces herself. She's a slim, dark-haired woman with an odd, not unpleasant speech defect. They are running all the tests again. Dan's had an MRI and an EEG that morning; a spinal tap is scheduled for the afternoon.

The room is light enough, with a large window overlooking the street five stories below. Dan's roommate is an affable guy on a Heparin drip after a mild stroke. He has the window bed but is seldom there; rather, he walks around, pushing his intravenous on wheels, trying to find a place where he can legally use his cell phone. I appraise him, estimating his discharge date, when we might move Dan to the window.

"Transport," in the form of a gloomy Bosnian, wheels Dan off for the spinal tap. I try to crack the hospital phone system. Our home number is in the same area code as the hospital, but it's not considered a local call. It has to be called collect, or the charges put on a phone card. Dan can no more negotiate a phone card than he can play basketball. On a floor of neurological patients, the hospital has made it impossible for them to call home.

Phyllis asks if we can do the admission interview. "Since Mr. Zinkus has difficulty speaking, I'll get the information from you, OK?"

OK. The questions are nuts-and-bolts stuff I can easily answer. No, we are not married. No, he does not have a Health Care Proxy. Phyllis describes several tests that Dan will have, such as one for vision that's neurological, not ophthalmological. The brain biopsy will take place as early next week as Dr. Ehrlich can schedule it; maybe Monday.

"Anything else you want to tell me, that I haven't thought to ask?"

"If you're doing all those tests on him . . . can you test his hearing, too?"

She smiles. "Maybe we can do that too."

Phyllis has obviously done these interviews before; she's careful and professional, but also friendly and relaxed. Her odd, nasal speech inflection is fascinating. My stomach unclenches one knot. Dan has a good nurse.

I never see her again.

Holly, the speech therapist, gives Dan a swallow test. I stop breathing while he takes a sip of water from a straw in a glass. She listens to his throat with her stethoscope. He makes no noise. She feeds him a spoonful of baby food and listens again. He gives just the tiniest cough. She shakes her head.

"I'm sorry," she says, "I can't recommend solid food."

Dan is staring at the jar of green baby food as if it's a soft-shell crab sandwich.

I arrive home to sixteen telephone messages. The appliance repairman is petulant: Why don't I call him? Dr. Ehrlich's assistant has realized it might be difficult for us to come up for the pretesting at 7 a.m. She can change that time, if we need her to.

Is she deaf? It's just five. I dial quickly, and, miraculously, get her.

Yes, she got my message from yesterday. "But I thought he might be discharged."

"He can't walk, he can't talk, and he's going to be fed through a tube in his nose. Why would they discharge him?"

"—I don't know about that. These tests are usually done on an outpatient basis."

Dan's mother makes sure to answer the phone when I call. "What did you think, that I couldn't take it?"

"—No, I didn't think that." What I thought was that she is so hard of hearing and I am so tired that I can't shout the details of these impossible days. "I knew Judy would write it down," I say.

And my mother. "Did they tell you what's wrong with him? If you didn't get the diagnosis today, you won't get it all weekend."

"They won't say anything before the brain biopsy on Monday."

"I really think you should put the dogs in a kennel. I'll pay for it. Then you won't have to worry about them."

"Why *won't* you let me do this the way I want to!"

I've never exploded at her like that, and she backs down. "I just wanted you to know that I meant it."

It's not only that I fear Dan would be horrified, more upset than reassured, if I kenneled his beloved Cooper; that I would miss the dogs; that my mother thinks it still costs $5 a day to kennel a dog, not $15, per day, per dog; it's also that this, this way of life, is starting to feel long term, a matter not of days or weeks, but months.

Saturday when I arrive, Jane and Judy are standing together alongside Dan's bed. All three of them look toward me as if finally the rescue squad has come. I kiss everyone hello, starting with Dan. I remind myself that I am not the rescue squad.

"Dr. Nason was here," says Judy. "He was looking for you."

Dr. Nason?

"The attending physician," says Dan's nurse of the day. "The one who *admitted* him," as if I'm an idiot.

"We never saw any Dr. Nason. We saw Dr. Damon and two Russian doctors. One of them was named Marta."

"Dr. Marta's just the resident. Dr. Nason is the attending."

I stand at the nurse's station, writing all this down in my daybook, trying to be responsible, an informed advocate. On the wall across from the station hangs a large plastic board imprinted with a grid and marked with a black flow pen. Each patient is listed by last name, with room and bed number, nurse and doctor. For Dan it's Dr. Nason. His name stays on the grid for the three weeks that Dan spends on the neurology floor, but the doctor remains invisible. A Dr. Koerner comes around and becomes the doctor of record. Dr. Marta does all the work.

"What's Dr. Marta's last name?"

The nurse laughs. "No one can pronounce it. She's known as Dr. Marta."

Dr. Ehrlich stops by, wearing another elegant suit. He will add Dan to his surgical schedule for Monday.

"He's so much worse than when I saw him," he says.

A nurse and an orderly help Dan into a sort of rolling Barcalounger and we take him, and his intravenous drip, a few doors away to the sitting area at the end of the hall. I'm starving and have to pee but Dr. Nason has said he might stop by this afternoon, and if I miss him again, he, and any information he might have, will be lost to me for at least 24 hours.

I'm out at the nurse's station, waiting until Dan's nurse gets off the phone, hoping that Phyllis will come on at three o'clock. The nurse finishes her call and keeps her eyes down, not looking at me, standing directly in front of her.

"Excuse me," I say. "Do you know if Dr. Nason is still in the hospital?"

"Yup, he's still on."

It's only my second day there. I don't think to ask her to page him, and she doesn't offer.

Jane and Judy leave at about two; it's their custom to go to 4:30 Mass on Saturday. Before they depart, I rush to the ladies room. But only the man from the TV rental company comes by this afternoon. Dan frowns when I pay for a week.

"The brain biopsy is Monday. They won't discharge you before Wednesday. You might as well have TV.

"Did you do your exercises? Let's do them." Holly, the speech therapist, has left him a sheet of facial exercises. There's a moue, almost like a kiss, and a grin, big and wide, and touching the front of his teeth with his tongue. He's supposed to do each exercise six times before going on to the next, but he won't, he does them in a series, repeating each series faithfully. We sit, making faces at each other; I giggle for both us.

Sunday I get to the hospital early. "You would have loved it," I tell Paul on the phone that night. "I come barreling around the door into the room and there, sitting right next to Dan's bed, is a black guy with a shaved head. Three hundred pounds. Street clothes. His job is to keep Dan out of trouble."

"I'm the sit," James tells me.

"—The what?"

"The Safety Companion," he says patiently. "But we're called the 'sit,' 'cause, we sit. We help the patient. He needs something, I get it for him. Like, we've been looking at the newspapers. He likes that."

"He does. Thank you for sharing your papers." James has brought the *Times Union* and the *Daily News*. I have our *Times Union* and the *Times*; Dan's half of the room is starting to look like our house.

"I'll go down the hall now you're here, maybe get a snack," says James. "But if you need anything, call me. I won't be far away."

"He seems nice," I whisper to Dan with a shrug. *Are you ready to take small comforts?*

When James comes back, over the next few hours, we chat. He works full time in the hospital, in maintenance, and lives nearby. He's divorced, and "sits" on his off-hours to make extra money. Dan is interested in him enough to test him.

"Dude, where you goin.'"

Dan doesn't acknowledge James's gentle question. He's making motions to get out of bed, on the other side.

"Maybe he has to use the toilet," I say, not believing it.

"Then I help him with the commode."

James closes the curtain around the bed. I wait in the sitting area, watching gray thunderheads roll over the city.

Later, we're all in the room again. The nurse has raised the bar on the far side of the bed. I sit next to Dan on the open side, with James no more than a yard away. The TV is tuned into a baseball game—finally, after all these years, Dan has cable—and I'm working my way through the *Times*. Suddenly Dan has the bar on the other side of the bed halfway down. Immediately James is on that side.

"Tryin' to get away again, huh."

Dan grins, lopsided, crafty.

"No, man, can't let you do that." James begins raising the bar. Dan keeps hold of it, pressing down.

"What? You fightin' me? You can't beat me." But James can't raise the bar. He's now clasping Dan's hand, trying, unsuccessfully, to pry it off the bar. When they're almost arm wrestling the thing, James says, "OK, you want to arm wrestle?"

Dan nods.

"Leave that bar right there."

James moves his chair to Dan's side before Dan can get the bar down much farther.

"I'll do it with my left hand, and I'll still beat you."

Another test. I watch in silence, barely breathing. Dan holds his own for a good minute. I hope he's happy with that. Probably he isn't.

At three, James is off: "Good luck, folks." And he, too, disappears.

I try to call Dan that first weekend, evenings from home. I take a deep breath and dial. I let the phone ring several, many times, knowing it's hard for him to reach it and hoping someone will help him. I have little in the way of news—just reassurances that the dogs are fine, a list of people who've called. I can't understand what he says. I might hear a croak or a whisper, but I can't make out the words. "I'm sorry, sweetie. I can't hear you. You can tell me tomorrow."

Sunday night the second-shift sit—a small, wiry woman without James's social skills—answers and gives Dan the phone. "I'll be back tomorrow morning," I remind him. "Dr. Ehrlich will do the brain biopsy tomorrow."

He says something I can't understand.

"Danny, I'm sorry you're there alone. I'm sorry this happened to you. I miss you and I love you."

"Good-bye," he says, blindsiding me, who can no longer understand him, if I ever did.

Monday, June 3, four weeks after his first bad run, Dan has a brain biopsy. I kiss Cooper good-bye and tell him Rob will let him out at lunchtime. Lulu and I set out with a full water bottle, a charged cell phone, a sandwich, and a dozen dog biscuits.

At the hospital I sign the form that says we understand the dangers of the operation and the horrors—brain damage—that might result, and we agree to it anyway. It doesn't matter that I'm not Dan's Health Care Proxy or his wife. The hospital needs someone to sign the form.

Friends call from New York, people we haven't seen in years; Paul must be putting out the word.

"It's Kate!" I say to Dan, and his eyes and mouth go to all Os. At McGraw-Hill thirty years ago, she and Paul and Dan were a threesome. Now she promises a visit.

At 12:30, transport—the cheerful twin brother of the gloomy Bosnian—arrives with a gurney. Once I see Dan to the operating room, I'm to check in with the receptionist in the first-floor waiting area.

The receptionist is a nurse in a white uniform, a kind, efficient woman who explains the process carefully, as if for the first time. I must stay here or keep in touch with her. She will inform me when Dan's surgery is completed, and then Dr. Ehrlich will be out to talk to me.

I find a corner seat next to an end table. Tracy, Dan's sit for the morning, comes in, looking around. I wave.

"Is he all right?"

"He's fine, Ms. Zinkus. I just wanted to tell you that I stayed with him till they took him in for anesthesia." Tracy is maybe 18, blond, and very cute. She rolls her blue eyes. "I called him 'Dan' and they thought I said 'Dad,' and they're like, 'You can't be in here! No family!' and I'm like, 'I'm not family! I'm the sit!'"

I laugh with her. He must have loved that.

And then, in a rare few hours of peace, I wait. Dr. Ehrlich's news will not be good; I'm in no hurry for it. I pray that Dan is safe and comfortable and then I wait, suspended, before the next phase of this. Twice I sign out at the desk, go to the car, and walk Lulu on the sturdy green lawn around the parking garage. It's not very interesting, but it is a walk, on a fine day in late spring. Inside, the receptionist tells me all about her dog, a cocker spaniel, and gives me an article about therapy dogs, which I read and return to her.

"Do you have tickets for the parking garage?" she asks.

"—No."

"You buy them at the main entrance to the hospital. Ten for $10. And use one every time you park in the garage. They never expire."

Around two, a handful of doctors drift in and talk to

families. No one sobs, no one groans; maybe their news is good.

The receptionist's next round, at almost four o'clock, includes me. Dan has gone through the surgery well. He's in the recovery room and will be moved back to neurology shortly. Dr. Ehrlich will be out soon to talk to me. I tidy my corner and sit up straight.

Dr. Ehrlich eschews the drama of appearing in his scrubs. He sits across from me and tells me that the brain biopsy has confirmed a tumor. Because of its location, deep within Dan's brain, it's inoperable; too much of the brain would have to be removed along with the tumor. This means some kind of combination of chemotherapy and radiation. The oncologist will discuss that with me. The biopsy now goes to pathology for further study; a final diagnosis won't be available for at least a week.

I don't sob, I don't groan. The only real news, the heartbreaking disappointment, is that the tumor is inoperable. I wish mightily that somehow Dr. Ehrlich were wrong. That pathology will say something different.

I make my calls. Can you hear me, I say. Inoperable, I say. Chemo. Radiation.

"Was he human at least?" Paul asks about Ehrlich.

"Yeah," I say, thinking. "He was human."

Dan is moved to 558, a mini ICU on the neurology floor with its own nurse's station. I come though the door to see him half rising from the bed, under the only bright light in the room. His brow is creased, his face strained, as he reaches up with his right hand, his arm extended as far as possible, a living parable of agony. On either side of him stands a nurse in white, trying to calm him, to press him gently back into bed, but he is strong, insistent.

"He wants his TV," I say. Over each bed hangs a small TV on a metal arm.

Oh. Their shoulders sag with relief. I kiss Dan's forehead while one of them fiddles with the dials. "We'll fix you up sweetie, but try to rest." He doesn't look at me, only toward the TV.

It won't turn on. Dan continues to try to reach for it. I go out to the main nurse's station, explain the problem, ask for repair.

"We don't handle that," the receptionist says, not unkindly, "and B&G is closed now. Give me a minute, and I'll see if I can fix it myself."

After an interminable five minutes she comes in, fiddles with the back of the TV, and it goes on. Dan lies back.

I'm as grateful to her as I am to anyone that summer, but like angels, these people—Phyllis the nurse, James the sit, and now this competent young woman—light on our lives for a moment and then disappear.

Anita and Rob have me over for dinner that night. Like Paul, Anita is urging me to get a second opinion, specifically a "record review" from Memorial Sloan-Kettering, where she worked for several years in public relations. Separately, she and Paul have gone online and come up with the same information: a brilliant young neuro-oncologist, Dr. Sheila Symington, will review a patient's records and render an opinion, without the necessity of transporting the disabled patient to New York. I'm already at critical mass, and I have no idea as to how to get copies of Dan's records out of the maw of Albany Medical Center and into the black hole of Memorial Sloan-Kettering, but I know I should do this. I should get a second opinion, even just to be reassured that we're on the right track.

Anita has written down Dr. Symington's phone number. "She'll have an assistant who will tell you exactly what they need," she says.

Dr. Symington's assistant answers the phone the next morning and dictates the information, sounding as if she will slay herself if she has to repeat it one more time. I'm to send a letter describing Dan and his condition and $300, and have copies of all Dan's AMC medical records—every test, every pathology slide, his entire chart, which is already the size of a magazine—sent to Dr. Symington. Once the file is complete, and only then, will Dr. Symington render an opinion, in about two weeks. A bill for pathology charges will come later, another $350.

I add that information to the red "Dan" file folder that I've started and head up to the hospital. Dan has been moved to a four-man room with its own nursing station. In the bed directly across from his is a thin, ageless man who seems to have had about a third of his skull removed. He wears what look to be huge round potholders on his hands. Next to him, in the one bed by the window, is a young man who also had some kind of brain surgery—motorcycle accident, I bet—and across from him, next to Dan, is an elderly man, barely conscious.

Holly, the speech therapist, gives Dan another swallow test—the enticing bit of liquid, the delicious baby food—and shows us, on her drawing, how he has failed it. He must, absolutely, have a nose tube or a stomach tube for nourishment.

"If you're having trouble speaking, Dan," she says, "I'll make a letter chart and find you a pointer. It'll be less frustrating if you can spell out words. Are you doing your exercises?"

He starts them: the moue, the grin, the touch of the teeth with the tongue.

"Good. Remember to do each one several times before you go on to the next one. And don't do the last three yet."

He continues to do the exercises exactly as he wants to, including the last three.

"Does he often act contrary to instructions?" she asks me quietly.

"Always."

Matt and Julie arrive, bringing with them an aura of happy early retirement and cross-country travel. Dan's face lights up and he swings his arm out in the wide greeting of handshake that he's always done with friends.

Julie's a good hospital visitor, who can chat gently around Dan's silence. But she's the new friend and she'll say, in her mild Houston drawl, "Y'all visit now, I'll go check out that soda machine," or scout the cafeteria, or make a cell phone call from outdoors, leaving Matt sitting awkwardly next to this being that he once shared so much with—an apartment, a sailboat, bird-watching, movies.

Dan is still trying to speak. We put our ears to his lips. Where is Holly with that letter board? The cheerful Bosnian comes instead, to ferry Dan, in his rolling Barcalounger, to the eye exam.

"Let's go along," says Matt, and we walk behind the chair while Julie stays back by Dan's bed, as if we three were going out to pick up the Chinese take-out while she brewed the tea. "Always go to a test if you can," says Matt.

The test, to ascertain damage to Dan's eyes from cancer, is stultifyingly boring to watch, but I'm happy to sit quietly with Dan and Matt. Exactly thirty years before, to the month, we rented a houseboat together on Lake Champlain. Dan was married then, to Kirsten, and Matt and I all but lived together. Dan and I had taken one brief, icy swim in the lake; Matt and Kirsten had watched from the boat. Years later, when it came up once or twice, Dan was quick to clarify that I didn't break up his marriage; it was over long before we started to date. But the friendship, and the mutual willingness to risk making fools of ourselves, were there, just waiting for us all to connect in lasting combinations.

Later, back in Dan's room, the sit, a severe little woman, has the only chair.

"Could I sit there, please, just while our friends are here?" I ask. "You could take a break."

"I'm the sit," she snaps.

"She's the honey," Julie snaps back, and the sit moves.

Matt and Julie leave around four. I stay with Dan another hour, and finally I hear him.

"This is terrible," he whispers.

I do what I can. Wednesday afternoon I stop Dr. Marta in the hall, she looking exhausted as always, her brow furrowed, not unlike a basenji, and I ask her if Dan can be moved back into a semiprivate room. She says she will speak to someone. "You do more than a wife!" she says.

Matt and Julie return, with new earphones they've bought for the cracked disc player, hoping that's the problem after its hit-and-run. Dan pushes the buttons eagerly, clumsily, again and again, but it doesn't work. Matt looks miserable, cross with himself for having made things worse.

The elderly man in the next bed has some sort of terrible crisis, and the nurses pop Dan into his

Barcalounger as doctors hurry in from other parts of the hospital. We wheel him down the hall, out of the way. How I miss the affable roommate with the Heparin drip; surely Dan doesn't need to be in a room with patients who are so ill.

We know, all of us, that Dan is dying, that Matt and Julie will probably never see him alive again. We can remind ourselves that we're all dying, we just don't know when—Matt suffers from rapid heartbeat and has spent time in emergency rooms; our parents are elderly and frail; we've all lost friends to cancer—but this—this attack—is outside our experience. No one says, "X went through this, and he had a good remission for a couple of years."

I imagine hospital staff talking out of earshot: *won't make it till Christmas.*

These days, my daydream is that Dan gets well enough to come home. In my mind's eye he sits on our deck in a wheelchair, facing the field, the shad tree in the distance. It's October, a brisk, sunny day, and he wears his leather bombardier jacket and brown tweed newsboy cap. He feels the autumn sun on his face. A newspaper rests in his lap. Binoculars hang from the chair. He watches the birds flit on and off the feeder and the leaves flicker in the breeze.

Julie and Matt leave for the next leg of their trip. Matt shakes Dan's hand and gives him a brief, awkward, heartfelt embrace. Dan's back in bed; the bed next to his is empty. In the hallway Matt's eyes are wet; Julie puts her arm around his waist. They each hug me, hard.

I lift my shoulders and go back to Dan. I don't have to start home for two hours, and anything I say—*they seem happy. What a lovely retirement. I wish we had visited them. They love you. So do I.*—underscores *this is terrible*. And, *good-bye*.

There is one thing. "Has anyone told you the results of the brain biopsy?" I ask him.

He shakes his head.

What do they expect him to do? Lie there, day after day, not knowing? Surely I'm not supposed to tell him, but in his place I would want to know.

"This is what Dr. Ehrlich told me after the brain biopsy on Monday. You have a brain tumor. Because of its location, it can't be operated on. It can't be removed. That means chemotherapy and radiation."

He winces.

"—I know. But you're so healthy otherwise. You must be a good candidate for chemo, and I wish they'd get started. They're still working on the pathology report. He said that would take until at least Friday. Today is Wednesday. That's all I know. They haven't told me anything else."

There. No one told me not to tell him. If my information is incorrect, or misguided, I can't help that. He has no other reaction. I sit next to him for as long as I can, and when I leave, I remind him, "Paul's coming up tomorrow," so he'll have something to look forward to.

Cooper throws up his breakfast Thursday morning and at night doesn't eat his dinner. At the hospital, word comes from the nursing manager that Dan is not to be moved to a semiprivate room. "A nursing decision," says the nurse, a pleasant young woman with an accent straight out of *NYPD Blue* and a swath of chestnut hair down to her waist. She's reviewing Dan's chart with me, to see if the pathology report has come in (no), when she discovers that Dan should have had daily physical therapy since admission; Dr. Marta ordered it a week ago, on May 30.

"What kind of a nursing decision is that?"

"—That's a nursing oversight . . . maybe I can get somebody to assess him today."

She does. A beautiful young physical therapist, whose every inch radiates the prime of health, comes to Dan's bedside. She talks to him, putting her face close to his. She watches his range of motion, touching his arm or leg to guide him.

"OK, Dan, we'll see you in the PT room tomorrow!"

"That'll be fun, huh?" I give him a hug and a kiss, and he gives me his WOW look, all round eyes and mouth.

Friday Cooper doesn't eat his breakfast again, so I call our vet and we get an immediate appointment.

"Dan's in the hospital," I tell her. "It's hard on all of us."

Cooper stands on the examining table, blindly doubtful. Lulu snuffles the perimeter of the examining room, dragging her lead, looking for an escape route.

The vet can find nothing physically wrong with Cooper, beyond his being 112 dog years old. Depression, she says.

"Do something special for him," she says. "Take him for a walk by himself. Brush him, play with him—"

I'm staring at her the way I stare at the staff of Albany Medical Center.

"—I guess it's difficult," she says.

"Very difficult."

"—Do your best. Fix him something special to eat."

And that's how Cooper eats chicken and rice all summer. How I sometimes have an English muffin and peanut butter for dinner, but I always have enough chicken in the refrigerator and rice in the pantry. How I never turn on the stove for myself, but every few days I cook a batch of rice and poach a couple of fresh boneless, skinless chicken breasts. How in August, when I wake at 6 a.m. to temperatures already in the 70s, then, in the coolest part of the day, I cook the chicken.

And now I take both dogs with me to the hospital; no more favoring Lulu with a ride while Cooper stays home alone.

Dan is sitting in his Barcalounger by the bay window, accompanied by a robust nurse in training, a young woman who looks like she grew up on one of the farms still to be found 30 miles from Albany. Dan's had a shower, she says, and done very well, washing his hair and beard by himself. I report on Cooper's visit to the vet. They both listen attentively. "The doctor diagnosed depression," I say.

It's not this nurse, or any other nurse I've ever seen before, but yet another one, who informs me, briefly, that Dr. Koerner came by earlier and gave Dan his diagnosis.

She might as well have slapped me. "If I had known he was going to do that, I would have come up."

She shrugs. "The pathology report came in."

"—Dan can't speak. He can't ask questions. And I wanted to know. I've been here every day since he was admitted."

"He was on his rounds."

"I want to know the diagnosis."

She keeps her eyes down. "I'll get Dr. Marta."

So the harried Dr. Marta and I have another hallway conference, with me working my way through her accent.

Primary CNS lymphoma. Oncology floor, one flight down. Dr. Ann Moore, neuro-oncologist. But first—

"In CNS lymphoma, need AIDS test."

"What's CNS?"

"Central nervous system."

Primary central nervous system lymphoma. There. I have something to look up.

AIDS test. CNS lymphoma attacks AIDS patients. It's what causes the blindness, paralysis, eventual coma. For that reason, Dan's HIV status has to be ascertained before he can begin chemotherapy. If he has AIDS, his immune system will already be suppressed, and chemotherapy will be contraindicated. Instead, he would have radiation, which is already contraindicated because while it might hold off the lymphoma for a while, it is also likely to cause further brain damage.

By state law, Dan must give informed consent before his HIV status can be tested. That requires an interview. It's Friday afternoon, and the social worker who would do the interview is not on duty. Her assistant is, a woman in her twenties who has held her job for a week. This woman, in a dress, pumps, and nylons that shout *first job*, talks to Dan, but because of her lack of experience, with him or anything else, she cannot be confident that he understands her. I can't be present to help because by law, the patient must be interviewed alone. She is sorry, but the interview and signoff will have to wait until Monday, when her supervisor returns. This postpones the blood draw for the test and the results of the test, which take a week in any case.

The immune system, I say that night on the phone. They can't give chemo to a suppressed immune system.

"But he's always been so . . . loyal," says my mother, the only one to voice the thought. In fact, he hasn't been, but among all my worries, AIDS isn't prominent.

"If only he had AIDS," says Josh. "They'd give him the cocktail and a fistful of condoms and send him home."

It's Saturday, and I've arrived at the hospital to find Dan surrounded by friends—Josh and Cathy, whose wedding we attended twenty years ago; Kate, from his McGraw-Hill days; and Tom and Gene, his friends from high school. With Tom, Dan canoed the length of the Connecticut River, weekends, over the course of two years. Two months ago, in April, they started this season's day hikes.

Cathy and Josh have decided that the theme of the day is ducks. Dan wears a new baseball cap with a yellow duck on the front, and a small yellow duck sits on his bedside table. He looks a little goofy, not a look he's ever cultivated, but "Dan happy" is the note in my daybook for June 8. I'm happy, too, even though it's too much like a party here, with not enough time to give everyone the attention they deserve, and I wish I could somehow orchestrate visits, so that we're not an open house one day and deserted on the next. But this hospital is three hours north of New York and two hours west of Worcester, where Tom and Gene live. I feel lucky anyone comes at all.

I also feel lucky that Kate, a hospital volunteer in the city, hasn't brought the candy she promised—"you leave it in the room, and then the nurses come by a lot, to get a piece of candy, and they pay attention to him," she said on the phone yesterday.

"—He can't eat anything. He has a tube up his nose. It would torture him."

Was that my mistake? I wonder much later. Not keeping candy in the room?

Tom and Gene go out to the diner nearby for lunch. Cathy and Kate have both brought boom boxes and tapes—Kate, music, and Cathy, books. Dan chooses Cathy's tape of *Grendel*, the Seamus Heaney translation of the Beowulf legend—"it's really scary," she promises—and Kate sets up her player and helps Dan put on the earphones. He puts his duck hat back on over them. Tom and Gene return from lunch. Dan sits in his bed, earphones on. I can't believe he's really following the tape. Is he mocking us? Or being polite, trying to show his appreciation. Kate leaves to catch the train back home. I walk her to the elevator.

"I know Dan doesn't care, but I will pray for him, and for you," she says.

"I care. Pray for us."

Tom and Gene leave soon afterward. I hug them, relieved at how quickly they've come. The summer stretches ahead. Gene's teaching duties will end; Tom, a lawyer, might have a lighter caseload. I imagine their wives visiting with them; over the years, we've been six many times. Tom's two sons grew up with Dan as a virtual uncle; surely they'll come too.

They don't, not any of them, not ever. I put Tom on my e-mail update list; he sends Dan a postcard from a car trip they take. He calls after that, talking mostly about the trip. *He's trying to treat me like a normal person.* But I'm not a normal person, I'm the heartbroken mate of his oldest friend. Maybe I should have asked: *he'd be so happy to see you.* Instead, I remind myself, *people do what they can.* I remind myself that the rest of our friends are extraordinary, helping with dozens of details. If a handful breaks my heart, well, isn't that the way of the world. You can't ask people to be kind to you.

Sonia, who used to call Dan daily for advice, doesn't break my heart. Now she calls me, weekly, explaining why she can't visit. Her mother is sick. Her father is sick. She fell off a ladder and has eight stitches in her head.

Whatever. "I'm sure you'll get there as soon as you can."

That Saturday, Cathy and Josh leave last. Dan and I look through Kate's music tapes, which offer little of the originality or edge that he likes. He finally taps something, and I help him set it up.

I go to the washroom and on my way back, I walk the length of the hall. The name of each patient's doctor is posted outside their room. Dr. Ann Moore has several patients on this hall. Ann Moore. A solid name, one implying clear speech and eye contact. My hopes inch up. She'll be in on Monday. We'll meet her then.

The motorcycle-accident patient is visited by a blond woman in her forties, apparently his mother, and a boy and girl in their early teens—siblings? The woman makes a point of showing the nurse the waterless shampoo she has brought. She's a nurse's aide at the Saratoga hospital, she says a couple of times; they use this stuff there, and it's really good.

I'm tired by then and wish they would keep their voices down, but I have to sympathize; that's why he hasn't had any visitors all week. She lives an hour away, has a demanding job and two other kids. How do people cope?

By offering shampoo. It seems overly fastidious, meant only to make up for her absence, but a week later I'm searching CVS for the same thing, wishing I had eavesdropped more carefully. I finally find No-Rinse shampoo, at $15 a bottle, half the money I have with me. I put it back on the shelf, walk away, circle around it, come back. At the hospital, the nurse seems pleased to see it and says she will be sure to pass the word along.

On Sunday Josh, a city guy unfamiliar with gas mowers, "mowed all the lawns with the hand mower," I report to Dan.

He gives me a look like, *what is he, crazy*?

"No, it was fine. Cathy bagged the clippings and I put them on the tomatoes—"

No. No food. No fun without you.

That night I write to Dr. Symington at Memorial Sloan-Kettering, describing Dan and his symptoms and promising that all his records will follow shortly, direct from AMC. I enclose the $300 consultation fee, which I've pulled together by getting Dan's permission to deposit his last check from *Time* into our one joint account, for this purpose. I thank Dr. Symington in advance for her attention and send my envelope priority mail.

They offer me money, our friends. Paul, Matt, Cathy and Josh. They sit me down at a table, their kind, intelligent faces reflecting years of education, decades of work. They have cleared this with their spouses; everyone is in agreement. A power of attorney can take time, they say. A bridge loan, they say. Matt knows I've always run things close to the bone. Glancing over my shoulder at the produce market on Sunday, Josh can see my checkbook balance at $200. For me that's good, a week away from payday; his balance has probably never been that low. Dan loaned Paul money once when he needed it, and Paul paid him back. These things happen among friends.

Because Dan worked at home, he paid the bills and then took his tax deductions for a home office. I made the payments on the home equity line that I had taken so we could do some renovations. I bought the groceries and made monthly payments into our joint savings account. Other than the house, the equity line, and a credit card we can both sign, our finances are separate. We have three cars—his idea—two of which are registered in my name. This month I pay the required bills, cut bait with our cleaning lady, and send $100 each to the three credit cards—his, mine, and ours—that collectively have a balance of about $3,000.

I thank our friends. If I don't have the power of attorney by July, I say, I'll let you know. To myself, I say, no loans. Go into savings first. A loan would turn into another bill, and then how would I pay it?

Ever since Dan was admitted to neurology they've been talking about discharging him. Shelley, the case manager, catches up with me one day. She's a heavyset woman in her 50s, calm and forthright, who tells me her job is to help me with Dan's discharge, whether he comes home or goes to another facility. In a tiny, windowless conference room, she explains that she shares this position with another woman, so that there's coverage every day. She must see the look in my face because she says, "No, really, it works. We keep our records in a central place, and we talk to each other."

I don't reply. She goes on. How does Dan get paid?

"He submits a bill. He's a freelance book editor. He does the work, sends an invoice."

"—*Oh* . . . OK, you should apply for his Social Security disability. Right away. It takes months to kick in. There's probably an office near you."

We talk more about Dan and his options. A rehab center will require him to take three hours a day of physical therapy, which he may or may not be able to do. A sub-acute care facility—a nursing home—requires less, but again, he must be making progress to continue PT. Otherwise, he's a resident.

Look into the places around you, she advises, just so you're prepared for anything. Of course we want him to go home. But no insurance will pay for home health aides; neither will Medicaid. You'll have to do that yourself.

Twelve thousand dollars in his checking account. A thousand dollars a week? More? Twelve weeks? Less?

We walk out in the hallway together. "You know," she says slowly, looking away from me for the first time. "He may get better . . . but he won't work again."

"Street smarts," says Paul that night on the phone.

"Exactly. Seen 'em come, seen 'em go."

Still, when Sonia says that their editor at Brady Publishing promises she will always have work for Dan, I don't argue. And I hold off talking to Dan's supervisor at Time Education. They're finished for the summer in any case; the job doesn't start again until September. They don't need to know.

"Caroline Knapp died," I tell Dan. "That writer we liked. *A Pack of Two.*"

He winces and turns away. And I stop talking about death.

Another cloudy, damp afternoon. I'm driving north on Route 9H, on the most active stretch of this two-lane state road, with off ramps, a McDonald's, stores selling computers or kitchen appliances or car tires. My trip to the hospital takes me across seven bridges, seven times when the hum of the road rises to a whine, and now I'm approaching the bridge over Kinderhook Creek. My driver's eye ascertains that I'm in a pack of cars, unusual at this time of day, that a young man (tan raincoat) and woman (red jacket) stand on the right side of the bridge, that they look not toward the water, but the road. What are they doing there, so close to the traffic? Will they try to cross?

Unable to see anything but the SUV in front of me, my peripheral eye on the kids, I'm the one who hits the turtle—"*No*!" with a great crack and crunch and a spray of blood that reaches to the passenger-side window.

They were waiting by the side of the road to try to rescue the turtle. Now some stupid driver has crushed it before their eyes.

I cannot bear it. But I have to. I'm in a line of traffic, I can't stop the car and break down. I have to get to the hospital to talk to some doctor or some nurse about something. Sobbing as I drive, I remind myself that Dan and I have rescued plenty of turtles, that last spring I carried a shovel in the car, so I could rescue a snapping turtle of any size by myself, that I remember Dan crossing our road, his arms extended, hands on either side of the shell of a snapping turtle the size of a manhole cover—its neck stretched, jaws open, ready to kill.

Now I have obliterated all those credits. I leave the turtle's blood on my car for weeks.

I'm sitting at my desk at the office, gazing out the window at the dogwood, now in full leaf. As long as I pretend to work half a day most mornings, I can get through this month; July 1, a new vacation year starts.

The phone rings: the social worker from neurology. Dan will be discharged soon, she says, probably next week. What am I going to do with him?

"—I thought Shelley was supposed to help me with that."

"Shelley's on vacation."

"—What about the case manager she shares the job with?"

"She's not in today. Is he going to come home?"

"—I don't know. I have to work."

"Sometimes people's families' help out. Take a day or two each week."

"My parents are elderly. My brother and sister work. They're not close by."

"Then you'll need home health aides. Insurance and Medicaid don't pay for them. You have to pay for them yourself."

"I know that. But I don't know where to find a home health aide."

"I have a list of home health care services. I can leave you a copy in his room."

When I arrive at the hospital that afternoon, an envelope addressed to me lies on Dan's bedside stand. In it are three pages of a list, in seventh-generation photocopying, of agencies that dispatch home health care aides. They're all based around Albany; surely no one they hire would want to drive an hour south, if they have a car, for minimum-wage pay.

Somehow, I don't worry about this. Maybe it's because I know Dan so much better than they do. I know how far, how fast, he's fallen. I know, in my own street smarts, when nothing's going well.

Or maybe it's because I have Maria to talk to. "I could take a day," she says, without my asking. "I could bring my laptop and be working from home."

I could probably take a day too, leaving only three to fill. Maybe Rob and Anita would take one. Maybe Ted, another retired friend, could take one. I could ask our neighbor Sandy if she could do a day; she's strong and cheerful and has done that kind of work before. I would pay her, of course, I would pay any of them, so that Dan could stay home with friends. I start to think, we can do this.

Later I think, it wouldn't have worked. Rob and Anita aren't strong enough. Sandy has a job. Ted turns me down when I ask if I can hire him to paint the porch; too busy, he says.

By then it doesn't matter.

Visitors come and go, "good" or "not so good." John, my stepfather, has volunteered for an agency that visits shut-ins and he can chat with a patient in a way that acknowledges his humanity without demanding a lot of him. My poor mother is terrified and perplexed, and Jane and Judy have always depended on Dan to entertain them, rather than the reverse.

I, as much as anyone, find it hard to talk to him. I can't come bustling into the room of a Saturday afternoon and say, well, dear, I sold the Jacob's Pillow tickets! No problem there! And I'm negotiating about our reservation in Provincetown! If they can re-rent that bayside apartment we liked so much, then they'll move our deposit to September. You'll be done with chemo then. We'll drive out to the Cape.

This I will tell him, if it comes true. How I'll get him out there, I have no idea. But if he can go, I will take him.

My note for Sunday, June 9, says "Dan unhappy" and he is so unresponsive, barely noting our presence, pretending to read the Sunday papers, that after my mother and John, Jane and Judy leave I say, "I'm sorry we can't do more for you."

He stares at me, the ugly, uncomfortable tube protruding from his nose. He has tried to take it off; the nurses stopped him.

Again, I do what I can, even if it concerns only real estate. The two young, hideously damaged men in the room are gone. I fear for the one across from Dan, with his vague look and the colorful mittens meant to keep him from damaging his hands, and timidly I ask Gwen, the nurse, about him.

"He's gone to Sunnyview," she says with her Welsh lilt. "They do wonderful work there."

"Gwen . . . would it be possible to move Dan over by the window, before someone else gets that bed?"

She thinks for only a second. " . . . Sure, we can do that."

"Thank you. It would mean so much to us."

And Monday afternoon when I arrive, Dan is stationed by the big window that stretches across half the outside wall. Most of what he sees is another wing of the hospital, but a swath of sky is visible too. A wide ledge runs the length of the window, where I arrange his flowers and cards.

I've been to the Social Security office in Hudson that morning, where I met with Roy, exactly the sort of pale, quiet bureaucrat you might expect at a Social Security office. He started an electronic file for Dan and explained that because Dan was 55, he could start drawing on his regular Social Security because he's disabled, *if* we filled out a magazine-sized form and Dan signed it in the presence of a witness. Even with a power of attorney I cannot sign it, or anything else having to do with Social Security, for him. "If he can't sign," said Roy, he can make an X."

Roy was very interested in the exact date of Dan's divorce, since Dan and Kirsten had been married long enough for her to receive death benefits, should she wish to. I knew that Dan had not been officially divorced when we started to live together, but that the paperwork had come through some time a month later.

"See if you can find the exact date somewhere at home," said Roy.

"—OK." A chore for the bottom of my to-do list.

Now, at the hospital, I'm on the trail of Dr. Moore. She works part-time, the nurse tells me, after the birth of her second child, and is in the hospital on Mondays and Wednesdays. This nurse gives me an office number for Dr. Moore and tells me I can connect with it from the hall phone. The number isn't the doctor's direct line but eventually I'm transferred to her office and her bored assistant.

"This is Deborah Mayer. I'm calling on behalf of Daniel Zinkus. He's a new patient of Dr. Moore—"

"She's in clinic."

"—If she's coming by on rounds today, I'd like to meet her. Or, I could come to her office."

"This is her outpatient office. She doesn't have an inpatient office."

"—She appears to have several patients on this floor. Do you know if she'll come here after clinic?"

"No."

"—How do I find that out?"

"You can call later, after clinic."

"OK. What time does clinic end?"

"It varies a lot. Sometimes three, sometimes later."

"OK, I'll call after three. Will you tell her that I called her and will call again?"

"I'll leave a message."

I go back to Dan, my hopes attacked but not completely dashed. "Dr. Moore, your new doctor, is in the hospital today. She's in clinic now. Remember clinic?"

He nods, remembering Dr. Ehrlich and clinic.

"She may come by later. It's hard to tell. Her assistant's a bitch."

He nods again, understanding.

Physical therapy cheers us up. There are not one but two beautiful young women in the PT room, the brunette from last week and a blond. They work with a group of neurology patients in rotation, setting one on an exercise and then moving on to another. They start Dan squeezing a ball, and by the end of the session they have him standing on his own, hanging on to a pull-up bar. He looks over at me, and I blow him a kiss.

It's after three when we get back from PT, so I call Dr. Moore's office.

Yes, Dr. Moore will see Dan today, but her assistant doesn't know when. Might be four o'clock, might be later.

"All right, I'll wait. What's your direct line?"

She gives me the number I have.

"No, that gives me the neurology office and then they have to transfer me."

"That's the only way to reach us."

I have both dogs with me so that I can stay late. I take them for a walk, tuck them back into the car with a biscuit each, and post myself by Dan's bed.

The room has a new patient—Evan, a man with a smooth, clean-shaven face and red hair that looks as if it's been cut with a bowl. Evan's chatty in a way both friendly and demented.

"Got a cigarette?" he asks me earnestly.

"—No, Evan, I don't smoke."

"Are you hungry?" he asks later. "I can't eat all this," indicating the half-eaten supper on his dinner tray. "Take some."

"No thanks, Evan, that's for you."

"You eat all of that, it's to help you get better," says Gwen.

"Not this crap. Dan want some?"

"Dan can't eat solid food—"

"—Sorry, man—"

"Thank you for thinking of us, Evan."

I try Dr. Moore's office again. Yes, the assistant snaps, Dr. Moore is coming, but she doesn't know when.

So I stay, tired and hungry and dehydrated and afraid to go pee and not wanting to complain to Dan. His sit that day is Marge, a solid woman with a bun of gray hair and a flowered smock. She's worked for the hospital for years, in various capacities, and these days, as far as I can tell, she lives here. I could ask Marge to keep Dr. Moore for the five minutes it would take me to use the ladies room, but I frankly don't trust her.

At six Sonia shows up, with Keith, her husband.

"We made it!" she says. "We've been driving around this stupid town for an hour. Why don't they put up some signs?"

Sonia is small, thin, a wired bottle blond impeccably dressed in this summer's casual chic. Keith is larger, with a shock of black hair over his forehead, and quieter. Sonia pulls a chair up to Dan's bedside and begins the narrative of why she didn't come sooner. It's Keith I ask to hold the doctor if she appears while I'm in the ladies.

She doesn't. It's six o'clock. Dr. Moore works late, says Marge. She might come at seven, or eight. "Go walk the dogs, we'll tackle her," says Sonia, and I feel confident enough to give the dogs five minutes on the lawn around the garage. Pushing them back into the car, I realize that the sun has shifted. It's starting to set now, with fierce rays slanting into the windshield. People are arriving for evening visits, filling the other parking places. The car will get too hot here for the dogs.

I return to the hospital, close to tears. "The car's getting hot," I tell Dan. "I can't stay much longer." He nods and squeezes my hand.

"Go," says Sonia. "We can stay till seven. If she shows up, we'll make her tell us exactly when she's coming back."

On Tuesday stories vary about Dr. Moore's arrival. Sonia swears, for the rest of the summer, that she and Keith stayed until seven and Dr. Moore did not appear. Marge insists that Dr. Moore showed up five minutes after I left. A scrap of paper is taped to Dan's bedside table on which the message "Dr. Moore will come midday Wednesday" is scrawled in sloppy block printing.

"Who wrote this?"

Marge shrugs.

I've met that morning with Glen Waterman, the only lawyer I've ever dealt with; he filed my will. We sat in a dark-paneled office, the door closed. Glen thinks out loud, and it was comforting to hear him plan things, to look at this from a different angle. He would write a letter to Dan today, outlining his need for a power of attorney and also mentioning the necessity of a will. I would pick up the letter tomorrow and bring it to Dan. If Dan agreed, then an associate in the firm would meet with Dan at the hospital and he could sign the form. Once that was done, we would go on from there. There was Medicaid to consider. Did I think Dan would come home?

"—I don't know. We would need help every day if he did."

Medicaid didn't cover that. No one did. What were Dan's assets? I listed them. Glen took notes. Who owned the house? We held joint tenancy. Was I sure? Yes. Could I bring him a copy of the deed? It was in the safe deposit box. I could have a copy made. Do that, he said.

He gave me exactly an hour, and I appreciated that detail too.

The hospital is another matter, and I need help here, too. I see Dan to physical therapy. "I have to talk to somebody, about Dr. Moore," I say into his ear. "I'll be back."

Then, feeling like a gunslinger, reassuring myself that probably I'll just make an appointment with someone, I find the second-floor Patient Relations office. When I ask for the patient advocate, I'm shown right in to the office of Gloria, a chipper blonde, carefully made up and dressed "corporate," but ready to listen.

I tell her how we got to AMC and as I speak, I realize that the problem is in Dan's admission through the emergency room. If his own doctor had admitted him, he would have one medical person associated with this hospital who was concerned with him, who oversaw his care the way my father did his hospital patients. Here, he's a theoretical problem, not a human problem.

"I try to advocate for him, but I don't do very well," I say, my face crumpling.

"You're doing fine," she says, pushing a box of tissues toward me. "Go on."

Now we have Dr. Moore, who isn't at the hospital every day and who is already overextended. "I can sympathize with Dr. Moore," I say. "She didn't ask for his case, she was assigned him."

Gloria shakes her head. "Dr. Moore cares for our neuro-oncology patients."

"But he's very ill. His symptoms get worse every day while we wait for the results of an AIDS test. He missed a week of physical therapy because the nurses didn't see it in his chart.

He needs a full-time doctor. We have to have another doctor."

She shakes her head again, gently. "Dr. Moore is the hospital's only neuro-oncologist. And she practices here part-time. She is an excellent doctor."

"That doesn't help if she isn't here. Her assistant is obnoxious. No one can even give me the correct phone number for her office."

"It's a new set-up, there are still some kinks."

"That's not my problem."

"—Let's take it from here," says Gloria. "What can we do for you?"

"I want an appointment with Dr. Moore. I know she's busy, but I'm busy too. I drive an hour each way to this hospital. I'm here every day. I can make myself available to her. But she has to meet me a quarter of the way. She has to tell me when she's coming and she has to stick to it."

Gloria nods, making a note. "What else."

"—I'd like to get a second opinion from a doctor in New York." I describe the record review process, what I need sent to the doctor at Memorial Sloan-Kettering. Gloria makes another note, nodding again, as if she knows what I'm talking about.

"What else?"

"—I think that's all for now."

She gives me her card—"come back anytime—" and a handful of complimentary tickets to use at the parking garage. I accept this bribe without hesitation; they'll make my parking tickets last longer. I leave feeling better. The rest of the staff will hate me, but they already do, and now maybe I have one ally.

Dan's still in physical therapy, sitting in a line of patients in wheelchairs, squeezing a rubber ball. He turns toward the door as I enter.

"Well, he knows you!" says the therapist, pleased.

Of course he does. I kiss his cheek and sit off to the side.

I love going to PT with Dan. Once, we ran local foot races together. Now I watch, fascinated, as they start work on the pivot he needs to learn for transfer between bed and chair. He has two running trophies at home. I should bring them in, put them among his flowers. They would see he's not an old, helpless man; he's a runner, he did well, he won prizes.

Today he has the chestnut-haired nurse again, the one who should be a dialogue coach for *NYPD Blue*. When she comes to PT for him, Gloria has talked to her.

"I can help you with all that," she says, about the record review. And, "You know, if you have a problem, go to the nurse first. Always go to the nurse."

"I never see the same nurse twice."

She nods. "Lack of continuity of care. It's the most frequent patient complaint."

"I bet."

"I'm his nurse for the rest of the week. I'll call Dr. Moore's office. You're moving him to New York?"

She calls Dr. Moore's office and contacts the various hospital departments about sending Dan's records to Memorial Sloan-Kettering. She tells me Dr. Moore will meet me at Dan's bedside tomorrow at 1 p.m.

And that's it for the chestnut-haired nurse. I don't see her again that week, or any other.

If there's any continuity to our stay at Albany Medical Center it's Holly, the speech therapist. Even late in June, when it becomes evident that speech therapy is too advanced a concept for Dan, she tells me that should his condition improve, she will be back. In the meantime, her goal is to keep him from becoming frustrated with trying to communicate. She decides the letter board is too complex for him now—*no, really, it's not, let him try*—and returns with a new manila file folder. The interior of this one is pasted with rows of small, simple pictures, each with one word underneath it: "radio" with earphones, "book," toilet," a clock with the words "what time is it?" Dan takes the folder and his chrome pointer and taps on "book."

"Would you like a book, sweetie?"

He nods.

"I'll go to the library. A mystery, maybe, something with a strong plot?"

He nods.

I can't believe he can read a book, but at our local library I borrow two hardcover mysteries with fairly large print, and I bring in Barbara Ehrenreich's *Nickel and Dimed*, which he bought for himself just before he got sick. They remain untouched on his window ledge, but they're comforting, stacked among his cards, which I rotate, standing up the latest ones; a cup with green swabs sticking out of it, like delectable lime lollipops; and no fewer than six vases of flowers. His apartment.

I hold off bringing in his footrace trophies. I'll wait till he's settled in oncology, use them as inspiration as he gets better.

We do get a medical visit that Tuesday, June 11, by the man I think of Young Dr. Andrews, a resident in gastroenterology. He's a soft-spoken, bespectacled strawberry blond, who's there to pitch us about the stomach tube. Once in, the stomach tube is painless, short, and relatively invisible, unlike the obnoxious nose tube that Dan keeps trying to remove. A stomach tube allows for better nutrition, which Dan will need during chemotherapy. If after chemo he can eat solid food, the tube can easily be removed. If he needs it again later, it can be reinserted, in a simple, minor operation.

"Do you have any questions?" Dr. Andrews asks Dan.

The head of Dan's bed is raised so that he's almost sitting up. He's still using his letter chart and chrome pointer. He spells out, W.H.E.N.C.A.N.I.G.O.H.O.M.E.

Dr. Andrews flinches. "That's not for me to say," he says gently. "I'm here from the gastroenterology department. We want—we need, to insert a tube in brief surgery that doesn't require a general anesthesia . . ."

He describes the whole thing again. "Talk it over," he says. "I'll check in with you tomorrow."

"What do you think?" I say.

Dan looks away, out the window.

"I found him persuasive," I say. "You won't feel it, the way you do the nose tube. You won't see it. You'll get better nutrition. You need to be strong for chemo."

He looks doubtful, still at *no. No permanent tubes*.

Does he want chemotherapy at all? We never ask him, this man who had to be force-fed something as benign as a vitamin. We just go ahead as if he agrees. I think he does. I think that's why he never signed a Health Care Proxy. He was afraid of someone—me—pulling the plug.

Dr. Andrews calls that evening. He apologizes for bothering me at home, unaware that I'm thrilled by the attention.

"What do you think about the stomach tube?" he asks.

"—You've sold me."

He will schedule the brief operation then, for midday tomorrow, and come by in the morning with the release.

—So soon? Shouldn't we . . . ? *No. There is nothing to wait for.*

On Wednesday I leave a message at my office that Dan is scheduled for surgery. I pack the dogs into the car, pick up Glen Waterman's letter, and drive north. I keep the air conditioner on in the car, even though I'm freezing, to cool it for the dogs. I've dressed carefully to meet Dr. Moore, in a black linen skirt and a white linen blouse with black trim that Dan chose for me last summer. My hair is overdue a cut but growing in well.

Young Dr. Andrews appears on schedule and gets a learning experience: if you have a difficult, brain-damaged patient, you don't give him the release form to sign. Dan stares at it for minutes, while we wait in silence, Dr. Andrews standing at his left, me seated on his right, Marge, stolid in her flowered smock, planted in a chair at the foot of his bed.

"Do you need me to explain anything more about the surgery?" asks Dr. Andrews.

Dan doesn't respond, just stares at the paper. I look away. Always he read everything he signed. I can't lead him. This is Dr. Andrews's problem.

"Do you agree to having the stomach tube inserted?" asks Dr. Andrews.

A flicker goes across Dan's face.

"He agrees," says Marge.

Dr. Andrews gives Dan a pen. "If you agree, make an X here."

Dan takes the pen, stares at the paper another couple of minutes, and then begins to sign his name. This takes an additional minute as his traditionally tight dollop of a signature wanders, wavering, across the entire sheet of paper. There's a space for a witness to sign, and he hands the form to me, tapping the space.

"Thank you, sweetie. Marge will witness it. Someone outside the family."

Maria arrives, with her gentle good cheer, having taken a day off for us. A nurse comes in to say that Dr. Moore's office has called: she'll be half an hour later than scheduled.

"Should we try to delay the stomach tube operation?" whispers Maria.

"Not for her."

"—Oh." Like me, Maria was brought up to respect doctors; this is new territory.

The gloomy Bosnian rolls a gurney in, and Maria goes along with Dan while I wait for Dr. Moore. I sit by his empty bed, my back to the window, uneasy. Never is it my intention to start off on the wrong foot with anyone.

Dr. Moore is fairly punctual and relatively cordial, and she looks like no one else in the hospital. Without exception, the other female staff members wear some variety of white pantsuit, like their male colleagues. Dr. Moore sports flowered dresses, a different one every time I see her, usually topped with one of a variety of pastel blazers. She wears nylons and colorful summer pumps. With curly ringlets of short chestnut hair and large, round blue eyes, she looks like nothing so much as a doll.

Dr. Moore speaks clearly and animatedly, like a teacher of young children. She is direct and take-charge without being bossy, and she is very good at giving me the bad news, usually in three different ways, without imparting any sense of panic. During this visit she describes the chemotherapy regimen. In addition to the standard clavicle shunt, a portal must be inserted into Dan's brain. Dr. Ehrlich will do that. Then weekly treatments will alternate, one week into the portal, the next into the shunt. This will go on for ten weeks.

"I know that sounds like a long time," she says, "but trust me, it'll go really fast."

Ordinarily, treatments are given on an outpatient basis, but because of Dan's condition, she wants to keep him in the hospital the whole time.

"His insurance will object," she says, "but no nursing home is going to hold a bed for him while he comes here for treatment."

I don't quite understand this scenario, but it doesn't matter, because I don't want Dan to leave the hospital either.

Dr. Moore hasn't given me any good news, which is fair, but when she asks me if I have any questions, I do.

"Suppose he does well on the chemotherapy. How much time might he have?"

"Oh, I've had people do very well on this treatment!" Her blue eyes are so big. "And they've had, eighteen to twenty-four months."

—OK, I think, I'll take two years. I'm new at this. It doesn't occur to me to ask her what percentage of her patients does that well, and she doesn't offer the information. Much later, I learn that it's probably five percent.

Dr. Moore leaves, and I head down to the second floor at a trot, to find Maria standing next to Dan, still lying on the transport gurney, waiting in the hallway for his surgery. I describe Dr. Moore—"little Orphan Annie grown up"—and our visit, without saying that we all have two more years together. Dan takes his letter chart and pointer and slowly spells out,

I.W.O.N.T.G.I.V.E.U.P.A.N.D.Y.O.U.S.H.O.U.LD.N.T.E.I.T.H.E.R.

"We haven't given up!" says Maria, looking straight into his eyes.

"We haven't given up!" I echo, mystified, taking his hand. Such optimism is unlike him. What—*the tube*. We are starting to insert tubes into him.

Dan's wheeled into surgery. The receptionist gives us a beeper so she can contact us when the insertion is complete. We walk our respective dogs—Maria's brought Argos, their chocolate Lab—and I show her where to park in the garage for a shorter walk to the hospital. With no picnic alternatives, we sit on a dog blanket outside the garage and eat our sandwiches. The beeper rings—it's been less than an hour—and we hurry back inside. Dan's in the unit's recovery room; the surgery has gone well. Maria leaves then, and when Dan is ready, sleeping, to go back upstairs, I walk alongside the gurney.

In our absence—less than two hours—Dan's bed has been moved across the room, from the window to its darkest corner, to the only station that can't see out the window at all. His flowers are bunched up at the end of the windowsill toward the foot of his bed; his cards are in a stack.

If you have a problem, go to the nurse first. Always go to the nurse.

A nurse I don't know is at the desk in the room, her head bent over paperwork.

"Excuse me, why was Dan's bed moved?"

She looks up. "The nurse manager decides where the patients will be."

"Is she still here?" Their schedules are unfathomable. "May I speak with her?"

The nurse checks, and yes, the manager is still here and will be with me shortly. I sit at the foot of Dan's bed. Today's sit—the happy wife of the cheerful Bosnian—is stationed between the two beds on this side, and there's no room for a chair between Dan's bed and the wall.

The nurse manager strides in, a tall, thin woman with the manner of command. Dan's bed has been moved, she says, so that one sit could cover two patients, by sitting between them.

"—If you had moved Evan over here and put the new patient next to Dan, then the sit could have sat between them, without moving Dan."

We stand in the middle of the room discussing patients as if they were pieces of furniture, to the backdrop of Evan's jovial calls: "I'll go over there, no problem!"

"He can't see his *flowers*," I say finally, and somehow, that seems to win the day. Aides are summoned and every patient in the room is moved, to get Dan back where he was and the sit between him and a new patient. Too bad. Should have done it right the first time.

I steel myself and call Dr. Symington's bored secretary at Memorial Sloan-Kettering. They haven't received my check, apparently gone astray because I sent it priority mail.

I don't say his name to the dogs. If I could say, Dan's coming home! Dan's coming home today! they would run around the house in their mildly autistic way and then come back to hear it again. Years ago, Dan took a two-week camping trip, and on his return, Cooper was so excited that he took a chance—and Cooper is not a risk-taker—and leapt into Dan's arms. Dan laughed and hugged him. "Good dog!"

Now among my worries is that Dan and Cooper will never see each other again.

The robust nurse-in-training twinkles at us one afternoon: "I've heard that four-legged visitors have been seen on this floor, and others may be welcomed." I'm as thrilled as if she had told me that Dan would regain full health, but Marge, the solid sit, scoffs. "Not on neurology. Too much dementia." She sees me sag. "When he gets to oncology," she says quietly, "ask the doctor."

Thursday I keep to a strict schedule of hospital in the morning and office in the afternoon. "Dan seems weaker than yesterday," says my daybook for June 13. "No nose tube, but it doesn't help."

Late in the afternoon, Georgia pulls a chair up to my desk. "How are you going to do this," she says.

"Just until he starts chemo, I'd like to come in half a day and take work with me half a day. Then I'll be back."

"You can't manage that. You look terrible."

Another verbal slap. I went to bed early last night after pressing this skirt. I think I look pretty good.

" —Let's try it," I say. "Let's talk again at the end of next week."

"You could take a leave."

"You don't get paid for that."

We lock eyes for a moment. "All right," she says, "we'll try it."

"Thank you."

About fifteen minutes later she calls me from her car phone. "Don't worry about it," she says. "Don't come in. Do what you have to do."

"Georgia, it's my job. I'll come in."

On Friday Dan has a clavicle shunt installed in the morning. I let the hospital do this minor surgery without my presence, and when I arrive later, everyone's in place except Evan.

"Had a seizure," says Marge. "He's in 558."

Late in the afternoon, while the staff is having one of their closed-curtain sessions with Dan, I go to 558 and stand next to Evan's bed. He's out cold, flat on his back, oxygen tubes in his nostrils, an IV in his arm. His straight red hair falls back from his chalk-white face. No more asking the nurse for a cigarette, no more sneaking off to the bathroom. Earlier this week a man from Sunnyview, this area's best rehab center, visited to assess him. He asked Evan where he was, and Evan thought for what felt like minutes. He seemed to be trying hard, embarrassed because he could not come up with the name. "You know," he said finally, "I've been in so many of these places, I can't keep them straight."

He never has any visitors. Maybe they come in the evening, when I'm not here. I doubt it. In tears I tell myself I cannot take on Evan, too. I ask God to bless him and I go back to Dan.

Saturday: the first day they let us give Dan water with the small green sponges on white sticks. Like the purple gloves, these sponges are so beautiful as to be delectable, their green the color of a lime skin, suggesting something tart and juicy and tropical. It's open house again at Dan's bedside. People come and go, greeting Dan and each other. ("Dan responsive all day," say my notes.) Friends sit among the flowers on the window ledge, their feet dangling. We dip the sponge into a paper cup of water, press out the excess along the sides of the cup, and give it to Dan to suck on. He does this time and time again, for the better part of an hour, clenching the stick with his teeth at a jaunty angle. Sometimes he reaches up, jerks the sponge from his mouth, and waves it at the cup for more. Other times we say, "Let me give you some fresh water, Dan," and attempt to pull the thing from his mouth with greater or less success. His face is stiffening, but his jaw muscles are still strong.

He's stopped trying to talk, and the letter board and pointer are only partly successful. Just as when we studied Spanish together, before traveling in Mexico and Central America, he will not simplify his sentences. Then, he wanted immediately to speak Spanish in the same articulate way he spoke English and now, too, he won't dumb things down. Instead of tapping out "M.A.N.D.M.S," which would let me know he wanted some M&Ms, his favorite candy, he taps out I.W.O.U.L.D.L.I.K.E.A.P.A.C.K.A.G.E.O.F.M.A.N.D.M.S.

By 4:30 everyone has left. Marge is on a break, and Evan's still in 558; the room is quiet. Dan doesn't seem tired. I have to do this; it's crucial for my survival and his. I take out Glen's letter and sit on the bed.

"Remember I told you that Glen Waterman was going to write you a letter about the power of attorney?"

He nods.

"Well, he did. Here it is." I unfold the letter and give it to him. I wait while he stares at it. There is nowhere else I want to be. The letter is well written, explaining in one page the power of attorney process and noting that when Dan gets better, it need not be in effect. A final paragraph outlines the further need for a Health Care Proxy and a will and says that Glen will be in touch later about those.

After a few minutes, Dan nods and gives me back the letter.

"OK? Do you agree?"

He nods.

"OK. I'll call Glen on Monday. Someone from his firm will come here next week with papers for you to sign. OK?"

He nods.

"Thank you, sweetie." I stand up so I can put my arms around him and lean down to kiss him on the lips. He draws me in. All summer he likes to kiss, long and deep and slow, drawing in and not letting go, holding me with his lips for minutes at a time. In some ways, like the rest of him, the kiss is "off," but I hang on. He's always been a great kisser, but it's been . . . forever . . . winter, in the kitchen . . . does he remember?

On Sunday we're looking at the papers. Behind me, my brother and his wife arrange mammoth pink peonies from their garden in a glass vase. Evan's back, sitting up in bed, talking away to anyone, listening or not, as if he had never left.

We've learned to prop the newspaper against the tray table that slides across Dan's bed. Today he turns the pages awkwardly, with his right hand. The left lies flat, immobile, alongside him. I lay my hand on it.

"You don't use this anymore?"

He looks at me as if to say, *obviously*.

Judy, Dan's sister, is canceling a trip to San Francisco because of his illness and wants to collect on her trip insurance. She has a form, with a Post-It note and a self-addressed stamped envelope, for Dr. Koerner.

"I thought since you're here every day, you could drop this off for me," she says.

I feel like I cannot do one single thing more in this

life, but she's right. I'm here. She's not. I wish they'd come more, help me cover weekdays, make their visits more than methodical, but I can't transform this family into something it's not. She takes care of their mother. I put her form in my purse.

Dr. Koerner. Once this month I catch up with him on his rounds. He has a long, slightly equine face, and he looks at me across Dan's bed, raising his eyes without lifting his head, as if he were dealing here with two brain-damaged people.

"A few days more before he starts chemo won't matter," he says.

"His symptoms get worse every day, He's lost the use of his left side."

"Any tiny change in the tumor can affect him, one way or the other, from day to day."

"Then doesn't he need to start chemo right away?"

On Monday, Dan is scheduled to have the brain portal inserted at 1:30 p.m. I work at home in the morning and then the dogs and I head for the hospital. I'll have time to see him beforehand and walk him down to the operating room.

Wrong. His space by the window is empty; even his bed has disappeared. Some of his flowers are in the trashcan. The cards and photos are gone, his locker is empty, everything stuffed clumsily into two plastic bags and stored in a closet at one end of 558, the mini-ICU.

Dan went into the operating room at 6:30 a.m. and is now in the recovery room, says the nurse. "We told you the schedule could be changed," she adds, in a cheerful reprimand.

In fact, no one told me that, nor did anyone tell me

to call at five o'clock in the morning to check on the schedule; otherwise, I would have done it.

While I wait for Dan, I track down Dr. Koerner's office, on the second floor, and explain to a young woman there about Judy's need for Dr. Koerner's signature for her trip insurance. I point out the self-addressed, stamped envelope for its mailing.

"I don't know anything about his in-hospital patients," she says with a shrug. "This is his outpatient office."

"Where is his in-patient office?"

"I don't know. I just work with outpatient."

"—This form is important to the patient's sister. How can I get it to Dr. Koerner."

"Put it over there. That's his mail."

Do I have time to walk the dogs? I check 558 first, and there's Dan, out cold on his back in a bed across from the nursing station.

"Hey, sweetie, you're back! I'm sorry I wasn't here. They didn't tell me." He has a new patch on his forehead, and Gwen, the Welsh nurse, says his temperature is 103. I pull a chair over. But his bed is high and all four gates are up around him, so I stand to see him better, and I notice a red spot in the middle of his nightgown. I reach out and touch it. Wet. I looked at my fingers. Blood. I look right, to the nurse's station; Gwen is deep in conversation over some papers with a male nurse's aide. I walk to the desk.

"Excuse me—Dan's bleeding." I hold my hand out toward her.

She jumps up, on the run. She lifts Dan's nightgown. "Ach, his stomach tube's out."

They pull the curtains around his bed and I move to the sitting area down the hall, from where I can't see the doorway to 558. Monday, June 17. The tube's been in only since Wednesday, June 12. Not enough time for easy reinsertion. What will they do?

Gwen inserts a catheter tube to hold the hole open and Dr. Andrews schedules a reinsertion of the stomach tube. At five o'clock I get in long enough to kiss Dan good-bye. He's still out cold.

I drive home through heavy evening traffic, sad and distracted, my eyes wet. Cooper whines from the back seat, pacing blindly, and I haven't the energy to reassure him.

Among my incoming calls this evening is one from Dr. Ehrlich. Just his voice—precise, unhurried, clean—underscores how unkempt—grimy and cluttered—the house is. He tells me all over again how they do a brain-portal insertion. They take a fresh CAT scan and use it as a map, without having any way to actually see where they are in the brain. And after all their talk of not using a general anesthetic, they decided Dan could handle it, which was why he was unconscious when I saw him.

There had been some cranial bleeding, Dr. Ehrlich says finally. They told me that was a possibility, he says.

"What does that mean?"

It could mean a number of things, he says. Including brain damage. But we don't know that yet. We have to see.

Some nights, I don't call people. If someone calls me, they get the information. This is one of those nights, except that everyone knows the brain portal surgery was scheduled for today, and everyone calls. If I'm lucky, when I pick up the phone, it's Anita or Paul, Margaret or Maria, someone I can talk to.

In bed, I lie on my side. Lulu snuggles in behind my

knees. Cooper curls next to my heart. I can't think, and I don't know what to pray for.

Tuesday morning the phone rings at 7:30. Too early for my mother. A friend?

Dr. Marta. Overnight Dan had a twenty-minute seizure. It took them forty-five minutes and two doses of Dilantin to stabilize him.

"I didn't call you at 2:30," she says. "I thought, you need rest, I will call you now."

I skip the shower, leave messages at the office. I keep my eyes on the road. I'm frightened, but I'm ready; we've had nothing but losses here, every step of the way.

Dan lies unconscious on his back in 558, much the way I left him, yet different. This is not the sleep of anesthesia, of something applied, but a profound sleep that starts from deep within.

Dr. Marta is still on duty, pouches under her eyes. I ask my question: Did the seizure cause brain damage?

She frowns slightly. "The seizure . . . is result of brain damage."

Today no one asks me what I'm going to do with Dan when he's discharged. Today the pretty social worker says I can use her office to make telephone calls. She clears a place for me at her desk.

Jane and Judy arrive. My mother and John visit too, and I'm grateful for all of their company. We rotate times with Dan and with each other. Every three hours I sit in the sun with the dogs for ten minutes and tell them what's happening.

Only when I catch Dr. Marta alone in a back hallway, do I say, "You were right not to call me at 2:30." I want her to know she made a good decision. Unless my presence had been required, I would have been too frightened to drive up alone in the darkest part of the night. I would have just huddled in the bed with the dogs, worrying.

Dr. Ehrlich stops by. The brain portal may have to be reinstalled, he says. Jane, small and gray, stares at him the way Cooper might, her head tilted, brow furrowed. The doctor explains the approximate nature of the surgery. The older folks aren't following him, but Judy is. They won't operate again immediately, of course, he says. They'll check the placement of this portal with a CAT scan, and only if it isn't usable, and when Dan is stronger . . .

Dan isn't stronger. He's still unconscious when I leave and he seems less responsive than ever.

At the office Wednesday morning Georgia's look suggests that Dan is at his end, or worse; maybe her face reflects mine. At the hospital, Dan's back in 554, the four-man room with the nursing station. He's awake—I can tell—but he can't open his eyes. He wants to, but he can't. I sit at his beside—the bed farthest from the window—and try, with my right hand, to edit the "finances" chapter of the college catalogue, which is due into production. My left hand is in Dan's, his good right hand, which squeezes mine rhythmically, again and again and again.

I tell him what I've done that day, that the dogs are in the car, that the deck was damp again this morning. I say, "Today is Wednesday, June 19. Tomorrow is Thursday. I'll go to the office in the morning and come up here in the afternoon. Because tomorrow afternoon, you'll be moved to oncology. Gwen told me that—they'll have a bed for you tomorrow, on the oncology floor. You'll be out of this horrible place."

I'm sure he hears me, but he makes no response. I remember something else.

"We haven't been doing your speech exercises. Can you do your exercises with me?"

Eyes closed, he makes his moue. He stretches his mouth in his silly grin. He sticks out his tongue.

"Very good, sweetie," I say, trying to keep my voice steady as tears stream down my face. "We can't forget those. Do them whenever you think of it, OK? Everybody around here thinks we're nuts anyway."

He continues to do the three he does best, the moue, the grin, the tongue, over and over again. Reflexive? Exercising faithfully, as always? Or mocking me and my hope?

Thursday afternoon I walk alongside Dan's big rolling bed—a special bed, they've told me proudly, one that breathes with him—carrying his belongings in two big plastic bags provided by the hospital. He still can't open his eyes, so I describe our trip. The oncology unit "is the same, only different. Long hallway, nurse's station on our right. But there's no sitting area at the end, just a couple of chairs. The lounge is over by the elevator, without any windows."

His new semiprivate room is tiny; barely space for one peony blossom. It enforces the two-visitors-per-patient rule, I guess; otherwise, we'd be sitting in each other's laps.

Dan's roommate is Charlie, a small young man with hair that flows to his shoulders and a beard to his chest. As usual in the hospital, none of us has any privacy, and now this means enduring Charlie's whining, nasty complaints to his mother and wife, who visit regularly, things along the lines of, "I told you, whenever you visit me, bring a cup of coffee from McDonald's! Is that so hard to remember!" Over the next few days I remind myself that Charlie is ill, but it's all I can do not to pull these two women aside and tell them they don't have to put up with that.

On Thursday I sit next to Dan in the sliver of space between his bed and the wall, just wide enough for a bedside cabinet and a chair. He squeezes my hand rhythmically, again and again, and I begin to cry, as silently as possible, wiping my eyes on my jacket sleeve.

His nurse those first few days is Johanna, an attractive, olive-skinned young woman with a British accent. She comes into the room now and sees the tears rolling down my face. She leaves immediately and comes back with a box of tissues.

"What's wrong?" she asks.

What's wrong seems all too evident, and at the same time I can't admit that I had hoped that last night's first chemotherapy treatment would make any immediate change. She will see me as someone foolish, who expects miracles.

She stands, waiting for a response.

"I just thought . . . he might open his eyes."

"Aahh." She nods sympathetically and walks away.

Cathy calls that night from New York. It's 10 o'clock, and her voice is urgent. "You've got to get a power of attorney—you can't do anything without it."

"The lawyer is coming to Dan's bedside tomorrow. Dan knows he's coming."

"But it has to be notarized. You need a notary there, too."

"I'm sure the lawyer knows that."

"What if he doesn't? Is there a bank near the hospital? Can you go there on your way in and let them know you'll need a notary?"

"Cathy, the lawyer has done this before. That's why I'm paying him." I can hear the impatience in my voice, but Cathy goes on about the notary, the paper, the bank, until we're shouting at each other.

"But what if he doesn't know!"

"Then that's his mistake! He'll do it over again!"

Friday afternoon, as I drive north with the dogs, I smell something bad. I glance back, to see Cooper having diarrhea all over the back seat of my Jetta, our "good" car. I can only cry out his name—"Cooper, Cooper, *Cooper*"—part fury, part sob.

Fortunately, we're near a parking area just south of the interstate. Fortunately, I've stretched a perfectly good sleeping bag liner across the back seat to protect it. I pull over, put the liner into the trunk and use paper towels to wipe feces off the seat backs. I walk the dogs and we settle back into the car. We're halfway to the hospital, past the most obnoxious part of the trip, the state route with its varying traffic speeds, cars pulling into and out of apple farms, the lumber store, the occasional home. All I want to do is sit next to Dan. But the dog is sick. In four days he'll be 16. I turn back toward home.

There I hose off the blanket and leave it in the sun. I cook a fresh batch of rice for Cooper. I let the dogs stretch out on the warm wood of the deck for an extra five minutes while I call Dr. Symington's office at Memorial Sloan-Kettering, to be told by the glum assistant that they've received nothing regarding Dan: not my check, not his records. Then I get into in the car and start north again.

At the hospital, Dan lies on his back with his eyelids at half-mast.

"Hey, sweetie, I can almost see your eyes again! Your eyes, your beautiful chocolate eyes!" I kiss his face all over, his smooth lids, soft eyebrows finer than mine, his forehead, cheeks. He purses his lips and holds me for a full minute, with his lips.

The young lawyer from Glen's firm is also a notary public. He's courteous and professional, talking to Dan as if Dan just happens to be lying in this hospital bed on this particular evening. At the same time I sense that he won't leave Dan's bedside without the signed power of attorney and he isn't going to spend all night getting it. For a few minutes, I feel safe.

Our annual AAA fee is due. We have "premium" for two drivers, left over from the time Dan needed some jalopy towed 50 miles. If I call AAA and explain that he no longer drives, the charge will be half, maybe less.

I can't imagine Dan ever driving again. But what if he does? And what if he discovers that I dismissed him as a driver? *You gave up on me.* I pay the full bill. For a miracle, the price is negligible.

Most evenings I call Worcester and talk to Judy, in conversations that never get any easier. She remains clipped and cool, without ever making the verbal move to end the conversation. I always have to do it: "Well, that's what news I have tonight . . ."

For all I know, she's watching television when I call and that's why she seems distant. But one night she's particularly cold, and I can't tell if it's just her phone manner gone extreme or if it's something I said, or didn't say. I hang up and am struck, as if by a bullet: *they blame me.*

There is nothing to do with this thought but get in bed and pull the blanket up over my head.

You shouldn't have let Kingston discharge him.

You should have gone to Albany sooner.

You should have taken him to Boston, or New York.

I'm so haunted by this that I confess it to Margaret on the phone.

"You couldn't have known," she says quickly. "Nobody could have."

And if that's the only reassurance there is, I have to grasp it. Guilt is a luxury when I have to get up every morning, take care of our dogs, keep my job, and go to the hospital. To paw our reality and worry it, like the dogs do an insect, is useless. Remorse can come later.

On Saturday Dan wears his glasses and his watch. He takes some interest in TV. The chemo is working! Monday he'll be zapped again.

Sunday I haul myself into church for the 8 a.m. service and in a kind of reward, Father Lauer is filling in for our rector. Father Lauer eschews the pulpit, preaching from the floor without notes, and he gives a good sermon. Today his theme is "God's plan" and it's as if he is speaking to me alone. The line of thought is simple—we may not always understand God's plan for us, but He does have one, and He is there, to see us through it.

Years ago, unable to endure any longer one of Dan's more extended depressions, with its accompanying fears and neuroses, I left him. I came back because I realized that with his wit, his intelligence, his usual consuming interest in music, books, movies—with most of the world around him—he was the person I wanted to grow old with. One day we might not be able to run or ski or swim in the ore pit pond on an August afternoon. But we would still have our minds, or, more specifically, I would have his mind.

Now Father Lauer is speaking to me, and I get it. It was my plan to spend my old age with Dan, but it isn't God's plan. I'm meant to do something else. It won't necessarily be better, but it might be.

People fight this line of reasoning: Is it God's plan that Dan, once vital and bright, is now frozen and brain-damaged? That's not the point; we're not the point. People think they're the center of the universe, and they're not. I don't have to thank God for everything that comes along, I just have to remember that there is, somewhere, a plan. The thought is exciting, in a way. Life is hell. And then something new happens.

Monday evening, Dr. Moore gives us a talk. She closes the side curtain against Charlie. She says everything three times, in three different ways.

When she's not in the hospital, other oncologists cover for her, on a rotating basis, week by week. The doctor covering for her last week thought Dan was in a coma because he couldn't open his eyes. The point of the story is not the lack of continuity in care or that doctor's idiocy but the fact that Dan doesn't have a Health Care Proxy. If we—Dan and I—want aggressive therapy and extraordinary means of revival, she will note it in his chart. Otherwise, he might not get it. Her language suggests that we should do this, that with the treatment working, we should go on. Dan and I look at each other and nod; just a second's motion. We look back to Dr. Moore. Yes, I say. Please put it in his chart.

She's right; we're down, but we're not out.

Tuesday afternoon I arrive at Dan's bedside to find Cathy there, up from New York for the day, reading to Dan from the *Times*. Our spat is forgotten; it's all I can do not to fall into her arms. Charlie insists we borrow the chair from his bedside. Dr. Ehrlich breezes in. He confirms what Dr. Moore said yesterday, that this week's chemotherapy will be a lumbar treatment, since the brain portal isn't usable.

"Why isn't it usable?" asks Cathy.

Dr. Ehrlich explains about the placement.

"Why didn't the placement work?"

He describes using the CAT scan as a map.

"Why didn't the map work?"

She keeps eye contact with him through this line of questioning, her head tilted in polite interest, hands folded in her lap, a slight smile on her lips. She keeps asking him why until he finally says, in essence, *we blew it*.

"Thank you," she says.

It's become evident these last few days that Charlie isn't fantasizing: he's been here a long time, but soon he'll go home. He's assessed by a variety of teams, including one to which he promises that he'll go to AA. He calms down with his wife and mother, and I start to sympathize with him. He doesn't seem to have a job, or a clue to what he wants to do with the next sixty years.

Wednesday, June 26. "Dan less good," says my daybook. "Does he recognize me? Rec'd first lumbar chemo."

Charlie's packing up when I arrive. "Won't see you again," he says. "Good luck to you guys."

"Thank you, Charlie. Good luck to you."

"All in God's hands."

"That's right."

I'm ready by then. I've spoken to three different nurses and one manager type with the same quiet question: "When Mr. Smith is discharged, would it be possible to move Dan to the window?" All four of them said yes. Three of them used exactly the same phrase: "No problem." One of them says it again on Wednesday.

So when I come bustling into the hospital Thursday afternoon and I find Dan in the same place while a comatose elderly man has the bed by the window, I am a minute short of murder.

My mother and John are there, my mother carrying a dozen sunflowers with stalks the length of my arm. "These are for you, she says. "Take them home. I know they're your favorite flower."

My mother has many memories of me that I don't share; this is one of them. There is no place to put these huge flowers except across the one empty chair by the bed. The sit's here too, between the two patients, and Ed, our doctor friend, stops by on his way to a medical ethics seminar.

Ed is very pleased with Dan's improvement. "Speech is next!" he says.

I know I'm churlish to be anything but grateful for that and for their interest. But if the new patient wakes up by the window, he'll think, naturally, that's where he's to be. For days. Or weeks.

I excuse myself and find Dan's nurse, the one with a peaches- and-cream complexion and Southern drawl—one of the "no problem" gals. Now she grabs Dan's chart and starts to review his day with me. A good report from physical therapy. Attentive when doctors examined him.

"I asked three different nurses, including you, and you all said you would move him to the window when Mr. Smith was discharged."

"—We forgot."

That's what she said. If it was a nursing decision to keep Dan by the door, so that he could be monitored more easily, no one told me.

I go back to Dan's bedside until our visitors leave. Then I ask myself how badly I want him by the window. Very badly.

Gloria, the patient advocate, is at her desk, nails polished red, jewelry in place. "I went through channels this time," I tell her. "I spoke to the nurses."

"Did you talk to Polly Naylor? She's the nurse manager, and she's absolutely wonderful."

"I don't know who Polly Naylor is. No one ever introduces herself to me. It's like *Going After Cacciato* up there."

She dials the wonderful Polly. Gloria's voice is low, as always, polite but firm. "His fiancée is here," she says. "He has to be moved."

Minutes later, back on the fourth floor, the elderly man lies in his bed out in the hallway as four women in white, including a tiny, bespectacled one I haven't seen before, work at moving the two patients.

Troublemaker. Tattler.

Too bad. They told me they would move him. They moved him.

Weekdays I wear the same five outfits in rotation all month until I have a day off on the Fourth of July and can get some more clothes out of the attic. It's a cool month, with regular rain; I almost look as if I mean to dress this way. Stepping off the elevator one evening I see a tall, pretty young woman waiting to get on. She wears the same worried, preoccupied expression we all do, and a T-shirt, gym shorts, and rubber flip-flops. *Summer. She thinks this is summer.*

On Friday Elliot sits me down in his office. How am I going to handle this, he asks gently.

I'm ready for him. "I'd like to continue coming in mornings and taking work home with me in the afternoon."

Elliot sighs. "It's been really difficult this month without you."

I find that hard to believe. My department is nothing if not overstaffed; the editors all do the same kind of work; surely people could cover for me.

But I need this job, and I'm ready with Plan B, one I dread, a plan I rejected immediately as too hard, a plan I was going to save for utter last-ditch.

"How about I come in every day from 9 to 4, without going out for lunch. That way I can leave early enough to get to the hospital in the evening."

"—OK," he says, still reluctant, "we can try that," setting me out on eighteen-hour days during which I spend three hours on the road.

I'm hurrying toward the hospital door that afternoon when I see a taxi leaving, with Evan in the back seat. His sheet of red hair, the chalk plane of his cheek, are unmistakable. I lift my hand, ready to wave, but Evan's completely focused on the car interior. He's bummed a cigarette from the driver—it's between his lips—and grinning, he waits for a match.

I take advantage of my last weekday afternoon in the hospital to speak to Gloria. Memorial Sloan-Kettering says they have received nothing regarding Dan: not my check, which I sent priority mail two weeks ago, or any records. Can Gloria help with the records?

"I won't be pestering you again."

"Don't be silly—"

"I have to go back to work. I'll come to the hospital in the evening."

"—That's too bad." Her face creases briefly before she recovers. "At least the light lasts longer now."

And then it's Sunday, June 30. Jane and Judy have come and gone. Dan and I have looked through the newspapers and watched the Marx Brothers on TV. Soon it'll be time for me to leave.

"Tomorrow's Monday," I tell him, "and I have to go back to work."

He makes his sad face.

"I know. I'm sorry. I'll miss going to physical therapy with you. But I'll come in the evening. I'll feed the dogs, and then I'll come up every evening."

He nods. What is he thinking? *Use my money, you might as well.*

No. He grew up poor, always worried about money. More likely he's thinking, *you're right, you have to keep your job.*

Albany, July

Monday, July 1. This week Dan will have a standard chemotherapy treatment, injected to the clavicle shunt in his chest. There's no operation scheduled to reinsert the brain portal, which means that next week, he'll receive a second lumbar treatment, in which Dr. Moore injects the chemotherapy into his spine. When I arrive at the hospital this evening, she's there, and I ask her why she doesn't just give Dan three additional lumbar treatments, for a total of five, instead of putting him through surgery again.

It's not as effective, she says. The short-term goal is to get him stronger and then try again to insert the brain portal.

Their short-term goal for me, then, is to put another release in front of me and point with the pen where I'm to sign, giving them permission to negotiate Dan's brain as if it were an unmarked country road, on which a wrong turn destroys not the vehicle but the territory.

I'm afraid to sign. But I want Dan to get the best treatment possible. Suppose I don't sign, and he misses out on something that could make the difference?

I push the fear out of my mind; no release yet.

We have our traditions, small things we do at holidays.

To describe them risks making us sound foolish. But every year on the Fourth of July, when the National Public Radio staff starts its rotation reading of the Declaration of Independence, we stop whatever we're doing, and we listen. The voices we've heard for years enter the house again, each reading a section of the sensible, stirring Declaration. Tears slide down my cheeks, and this year, by the time Red Barber reads, it's all I can do not to bawl. He was so long ago now, Red Barber; a morning voice in the river light of our apartment on West Fourth Street. Dan could listen without crying, but he was quietly moved. All those years of writing U.S. history for teenagers: this was what it was about.

Dan's nurse on the Fourth of July is Brad, an easygoing man in his early 30s, completely bald. He's the one who says, "Don't hold bowel movements, Dan. Just do it. We'll clean you up."

But there's no sit. I ask Brad about this, trying for a nonjudgmental tone, one that simply seeks information. He has to ask someone else, and an hour later he reports that with the holiday, and vacations, it's a staffing problem. The only available sits are assigned to a suicide watch "and that takes priority, obviously," he says.

I feel reprimanded and don't ask again for several days. But Dan never has a sit now and as far as I can see, neither does anyone else on the floor. Budget? I wait a week and ask again. And then again. I receive no answer, or its variant: "I don't know."

I've reduced the *Times* and the *Times Union* to their sports and arts sections, but I still carry them every day, in a large white tote bag along with my growing red "Dan" file. We look through the paper together.

"You know, he probably can't see well enough to read it," Dr. Moore says to me one evening, out at the nurse's station.

"—OK. But he's always read the newspapers. Since he was a little boy—he read the comics, with his father. I figure he can see the ads, the photos. He likes to track how movies are marketed during their run."

She looks at me, her round eyes big, more puzzled than enlightened.

The beginning of September, when Dan would start work again for Time Education, no longer seems a long way off. What he does for this ancillary publication, mailed to subscribing classrooms at the same time as the magazine, is keep up on the news daily, and then, in a few hours over the weekend, transform it into a ten-question quiz at a sixth-grade reading level. He's renowned in this context for his excellent quizzes, for thinking that's simultaneously comprehensive and fast. To go back to work there, he would have to be a completely different person by the end of August, less than eight weeks away. And Owen and Lucy, his coworkers, genuinely like him. I call Owen.

"—Maybe we'll line up a substitute for next semester," he says. "But the job is Dan's. In the meantime, I'll rent a car and Lucy and I will come up and visit him."

Silly of me to keep them from him. "He'd love to see you."

Would he? I never know whether his visitors comfort him, showing him that they care, or embarrass him, as they stand around the wreckage.

I don't bring in his running trophies. Even though Dr. Moore has him on an antidepressant, with his perennial tendency to paranoia, I fear he'll see them not as encouragement but an affront: *this is what you once were.* If I brought them in, it would be for the staff: *this is what he once was.* They see him as a sick old man. He is sick, but he has never grown old. He was in his forties when he won these trophies. He ran two months ago.

I do bring in photos—my favorite of the two of us, a close-up with our heads together. I look decent, and Dan's face radiates intelligence. Linda drops off wide-angle snapshots of the countryside in summer—bales of hay rolled, ready for pickup on a broad hill, the horizon a midpoint—and I rotate those in their frame. I leave the pictures on the window ledge all summer, placed strategically among the cards and a photo of Dan and Cooper that I took years ago. We had borrowed a friend's RV and gone out to the Finger Lakes for a long weekend. Dan was driving, I was in the passenger seat, and Cooper poked his head between us. The RV was large enough so that I could get a good clear shot of Dan and Cooper: their handsome profiles, Dan with the same kind of half smile he wore when he watched a movie, Cooper's wrinkled brow suggesting his perpetual concern with the driving, along with everything else.

Friday, July 5. Even with a day off for the Fourth, I know that driving home from the hospital at night, I'm a danger on the road, my mind shutting down behind my eyes, my arms and legs numb with fatigue. I wiggle in the car seat, shake my arms, and slap my face, but moments later my attention slides again. So I overcome my hostility to the local Dunkin' Donuts drive-through and buy an iced coffee on my way north. The shop is part of a Mobil Station and an Xtra Mart that were the first application Dan voted on as a new member of the Zoning Board of Appeals. The town doesn't need it, it's ugly— a windowless brick wall on an acre of concrete—and Dan's always felt bad about it: "You could look at their plans and not see that wall," he said sadly one day, apropos of nothing, as we drove by.

But desperation ends my boycott and five nights a week I pull in and wait, sometimes for minutes, for someone to staff the drive-through. I try to make a connection, to establish myself as a regular, but if the voices behind the microphone ever remember me or my red Jetta, they don't let on.

"I hope you're doing something for yourself to help you get through this—meditation, yoga . . . ," a concerned friend e-mails me during the summer. Well, something like that: I get through it doing my exercises every morning—a 15-minute combination of stretches and spot work that I've done for years—and I survive it on one iced coffee—small, milk not cream, no sugar—every evening.

Saturday night Margaret, Steven, and I go to a local production of *South Pacific*, the one show I wanted to see this summer. We have some vague directions and a map, and it's not quite dark yet, but we still get lost looking for the particular high school auditorium we're aiming for. Dan would have driven us there directly. Dan would have been annoyed at our lack of precision. We just giggle. And we get there on time.

On Sunday when I come around the corner to Dan's hallway, there he is! Sitting up in his Barcalounger, across from the nurse's station, not quite smiling—he still can't smile—but alert to my arrival, attentive to what's going on. Everyone is pleased with his progress, which is incremental but noticeable. He pulled his catheter tube out twice in one night, so for the moment—until the next chemo treatment—they've let him win that one.

"He was visited by the therapy dog this morning," the nurse reports, and I wish mightily I'd been here, to see if even a Labrador (not his favorite breed—too goofy, too needy) could bring him back to us.

"Did Maria come yet?" I ask him.

He shakes his head.

"She will," I say, worried that she won't, that something's come up. But ten minutes later she rounds the corner, at once glowing and steady. My joy is complete; I bet his is too.

"Hey Dan, you're sitting up! You look great! That danged Sunday traffic on the Northway—" she kisses him.

"I'll tell her the shortcut before she leaves," I say, and his nod instructs me not to forget.

We roll him up and down his hall. He peers into the other patients' rooms in a way that's not quite polite, but I'm happy that he's interested. We sit out in the lounge area near the elevator, and he watches who comes and goes. When the nurse says it's time for him to get back into bed, he helps them by doing his pivot, his eyes locked with mine—*see, I can do it*—and then, in another upgrade, we can give him the lovely green sponges soaked in tangy ginger ale.

Dinner that night with Henry and Todd, friends from church. Todd is a certified nurse's assistant at a local nursing home, and I'm hoping that he can advise me on care for Dan after the hospital—the good, the bad, whom to call, whom to stay away from.

Like Dan, Todd and Henry are superb avocational cooks. For the past several months we've traded hosting dinners, and at our house, at least, I felt the competition ratchet up every time. Their home, a large restored farmhouse, is everything ours is not today, tidy and peaceful, with every detail attended to. Henry's filled pots with annuals and grouped them strategically around the deck. I have him take me around and describe what's in each pot.

"Next year," I say, "you'll teach me how to do this." I have no idea what my life will be like next summer, and that's strange, and scary, a vast ocean without even a rowboat or an island in view, but it's not the scariest part of my life these days.

This summer, Todd says he's not familiar with other local facilities, or home health care agencies. "I only know my own place," he says, which is the county-run nursing home. It has a good reputation, but it's an old building filled with ancient people at the end of their line. I have higher hopes for Dan.

Todd does have information for me—a packet he's prepared, in a fir-green folder, about hospice. "They were a great help with my mother," he says.

I nod, thanking him. Back home I add the packet to the pile of newspapers and mail on the table. Monday morning, casting about for something to read while I eat breakfast, I open it . . . "Hospice: A Special Kind of Caring" . . . a pamphlet guide for Do Not Resuscitate Orders . . . within a minute I burst into tears over my cereal. This isn't us. We aren't there yet.

Wednesday evening Dr. Moore's wearing yet another flowered dress and new lavender pumps. In these duds she's given Dan his fourth chemo treatment, second lumbar. He's dozing now, and we stand at the foot of his bed while she tells me things she's said before—that he's more attentive and his eye movement continues to improve.

If he isn't attentive sometimes I wonder if he's bored, tired of being asked the same questions every day, but I don't say that. What I do take a breath and say, is:

"Would it be all right, if I brought our dogs—there are just two of them—to visit Dan sometimes? Only on weekends, when it isn't so busy here. They'd be on their leads, of course, and they're well-trained, there won't be any accidents."

Her doll-like eyes are full circles as she thinks. " . . . I don't see why not."

"Oh, thank you! It will make him so happy. Will you please put it in his chart so the nurse on duty will always know."

She puts it in the chart. She adds that he can leave the floor with family.

"Yeah, we had another patient, doctor let her dogs visit her," the nurse's aide with the funny twitch says later. "Right before she went into hospice."

Thursday, July 11. "You look nice and bright today!" says Georgia at the office.

"It's Dan's birthday!"

"—*Oh*."

I'm wearing a Hawaiian shirt that he passed along to me after it shrank—years-old soft, sea green, splashed with white orchids—and my fuchsia sandals. For a gift, I've bought him a book. It's stupid, I know, but so is anything else I can think of—music, food—and a book was the last thing he asked for. So I give him *Stardust Melodies*; once, he would have wanted it, and I thought it had more illustrations. In twelve chapters Will Friedwald discusses twelve popular songs, including "Star Dust," which I learned on the piano at Dan's request, "Lush Life," and ten others we love. I inscribe it to him—"melody of my song, my heart, my life." I find a card I've been saving for him—two insane-looking dogs on the front with a mélange of hearts and dog biscuits: "Ah, L'amour." "My dear Dan," I write, "I have loved you for 25 years! I will love you for 25 more."

I e-mailed a reminder that his birthday was coming up, and daily, he's received cards—three or four, five or six, usually lying unopened on his tray table when I arrive. Sometimes he wants to open them himself; other nights he seems satisfied to have me do the work. I read each card to him once, just to make sure he hears the words, but mostly I let him hold it and look at it. When a card comes from Kirsten, his former wife, he stares at it for a long time. She lives in Arizona now, and at first I think it odd that she's sent a seascape, until I realize, *she remembers.* She remembers that he loves the sea.

He doesn't seem very interested in my present. "I can read it to you, if you want," I say, but I feel he's frowning slightly, as if I brought the wrong thing. I read the titles of the songs, show him the illustrations that start each chapter. I read him the inscription, and my card; my voice breaks, which I hate: the sound of admitting defeat.

No kiss tonight.

While June stayed cool and moist—most mornings I woke to find the deck wet—July dawns as a perfect summer month, a kid summer, every day sunny, growing from warm to hot, days for the pond, the lake, the beach. More than once we stand in the parking lot at the office and say to each other, this is the best day we'll have all summer!

More than once I set off with the dogs on our early walk and watch the leaves flicker in the sun, feel the breeze pick up, and think, perfect morning for a sail.

But in mid-July, sometime after Dan's birthday, the weather begins to turn on us. *You like clear and hot? Here's clear and hot.* Nighttime temperatures move from the 60s, to the 70s and up (July 22, 10 p.m., clear, 82 degrees outside and inside the house).

We've never bothered with air conditioning. Neither of us grew up with it, we lived for years in the city without it, and this is the country. The house is surrounded by trees, and historically, only a handful of nights every summer are really hot. With fans we take advantage of the cross draft, drawing in cooler air at night, closing the house against the heat during the day. Now I want to leave the shades up and the windows cracked open for Cooper, and although Dan and I always slept with the doors unlocked, now I'm uneasy about it. But the house, with its few rooms and low ceilings, needs all the air circulation it can get, and by August, drenched at night, as restless as the dogs, I leave nothing but flimsy screen doors, one with a broken lock, between me and the rapist-killer of the woods; at least I won't suffocate while he creeps in.

Big surprise, I tell the dogs Saturday morning, big surprise! That's our code for "something very good is going to happen . . . later." It's too high-concept for them, but we always hoped they might learn it.

First I walk them, the ancient blind wanderer and the two-year-old, still with her puppy brain, each pulling and lurching in its own direction, with me between them. All summer I see myself like nothing so much as Lucky in *Waiting for Godot.*

Then we drive not north but south, first to take Cooper to the vet. It's occurred to me that maybe they can do something for him. Maybe he doesn't need to be crashing into the refrigerator, which has been in exactly the same place for twenty years. Maybe it's not necessary that he bruise his head against the door frames and that Lulu, meaning well, lick the cuts so that they turn into sores and never heal.

Absolutely there's something she can do for him, the vet says.

"She started with a shot of B-12," I report to Dan when I arrive at the hospital.

Brad, the nice bald nurse, is pouring the brown mush into Dan's stomach tube, and he nods approval: "That'll boost him right away."

She also prescribed something for his cognitive dysfunction, something for his liver, two additional daily vitamins, and a cream for the cuts on his face.

In the height of summer no one's coming to see us today, and there's no staff available to wait with Dan outdoors while I go get the dogs.

"Just bring them up here," says Brad, as in, sure, the dogs can come in the house.

I give the dogs one more walk on what is now tough dry grass around the parking garage and then, my breath shallow, making no eye contact, I hurry them into the hospital and onto an elevator.

Dan knows them at once, and he's glad to see them, even though he can't smile. He's a little rougher with them than usual, since even his good hand moves with jerks, but the dogs don't seem to mind.

"Are they as you remember them?"

He nods yes.

I'd expected the dogs to burble all over him, but the context is wrong; he's just part of a new place they're compelled to explore. I brought him one of his short-sleeved "vacation man" shirts, the cream linen one, which will go with any pattern of hospital pajamas, and his white newsboy cap. While I went for the dogs, Brad helped Dan put on these clothes and sit in his Barcalounger. We process into the small "family room" off the back hallway, me pushing the chair, Dan grasping the dogs' leashes as they strain to sniff the hospital. I thought they'd give us more to talk about, but they don't. They can't change our lives, our routines, which alternate the stultifying with the inconceivable.

Dinner that night with Stan and Katie: vital, white-haired, radiating the affection we've all shared for years. Stan is a retired physician, Katie a weaver and community activist. Now they tell me they're going to Los Alamos for almost a year, to housesit for their daughter and her family while they're in Spain.

"We'll be back next spring," they say, reading my face. And yes, in his late 70s Stan has taken completely to e-mail. I send him my updates, and he's replied with a report of their visit to Dan. But it won't be the same. I won't be able to share with them, for example, the disaster of Dan's record review by Memorial Sloan-Kettering.

"His what?" says Stan.

"You send his records to a doctor at MSK. She reviews them and writes her opinion, which gets sent directly to the family. Me."

"That's despicable!"

Then, I thought he meant that it was despicable for them to charge $300 and give an opinion on a patient they had never met. Later, I realized it was contemptible in many ways: a cash cow from terrified families in hopeless situations; a way to earn money while they looked for research subjects.

Twice a week, for the last month, I've called Dr. Symington's office and talked to her tortured assistant. They haven't received my check. They haven't received the records. They received some of the records but not my check. Is this the same Daniel Zinkus that lived at 285 West Fourth Street, who consulted their Dr. – in 1982? Yes, but we moved from that address five years ago. Our current address is on every piece of paper that's sent to you, but here it is again. . . .

They received all of the records but not my check. I fax a stop order to the bank, write another check, and send it certified. They receive the first check. I tell them to destroy it. They wait for the second check, which takes longer to arrive, because of being sent certified.

I make the dogs travel in their crates, an indignity they never suffered with Dan. Lulu falls asleep, but Cooper whines softly all the way, reminding me that it wasn't his idea to move to the country, that he is a city dog, happiest—*calmest*—lying at Dan's feet, observing the world from a sidewalk café, and never did he expect to spend his old age like this.

It's Sunday, and Dan has already sat up and is back in bed; this hospital never gives without taking away. I'm having trouble trying to get one wriggly dog to him while I hold the other. "Just put them on the bed, it's OK," says Brad. Astonished, I do it quickly, before he can change his mind, and finally the dogs can lick Dan's feet, finally they can begin to feel at home. Lulu rests by lying between his legs. She props her head against Dan's knee—she has always considered us warm-blooded furniture—her eyes at half-mast.

We're watching TV like this, me in the Barcalounger, Cooper settled under Dan's arm, when a short, stooped man comes into the room, preceded by the smell of stale cigarette smoke.

"Are those the therapy dogs?" he asks. "That visit the patients?"

"No, these are our dogs. They're visiting Dan."

"My wife would really like to see them. She's just down the hall. Can you bring them to her?"

The dogs are already disturbed, alert to the new smell—

"Please? She loves dogs."

—on their feet, pulling on their leads.

"Just for a minute," he says. "She just wants to see them."

Can't he see we're enjoying a family moment here? No, he can't: his wife is ill and she loves dogs. I kiss Dan—"we'll be right back"—and, praying that the dogs won't nip any strangers, I hustle them down the hall.

The woman is sitting up in bed. She has her hair and she can talk, but she's dying, her skin stretched tight and yellow over her skull.

"Bee-yoo-tee-ful," she coos. "Like little deeeer . . . " She wants to know all about them.

"Cooper is named for Gary Cooper . . . the movie actor?"

"Sure," says the man. "*High Noon*."

"Right. My husband named him. He could tell immediately that Cooper was the strong, silent type. Lulu's full name is Louise Brooks."

"Silent movies," he says.

"Yes. Because basenjis don't bark." Torn with guilt—we are giving them something to talk about—I time five minutes. "I'm sorry, but I have to go back to my husband. He's very ill."

"Thank you," she says. "Thank you, thank you, thank you."

With his right hand, Dan continues squeezing—our hands, if we're there, or the things we leave for him when we're not. A freelancer he worked with sends a pastel stuffed octopus—a mystery to me, why she would send such a thing, but it's filled with some kind of beans or grain, and it's good for squeezing. Maria and Judy bring him the hard rubber balls he used to strengthen his hands for rock climbing, and he likes those, too. I make sure one is always in reach, but as July wears on he moves to hurting himself, repeatedly slamming his right hand against the bed rail, so that when I arrive at night his knuckles are bloody, or by cutting his forehead with fingernails that are never trimmed by hospital staff. He's supposed to wear splints on his paralyzed arm and leg, two hours on, two hours off, to keep the limbs from curving beyond repair. He doesn't like these splints; often he pulls the arm one off immediately and shoves the leg one down with his good foot. There's something weirdly endearing about these actions, as he takes some tiny control of his life, but at the same time I know he needs the splints, and I wind up on the side of the nurses—"please sweetie, leave them on for just a little while." He pays no attention.

He also pulls out his stomach tube, which then has to be replaced.

I ask again and again what happened to the sits until finally Polly, the nurse manager, says, "He only had a sit when he was at risk for falling."

I stare at her. Feeling my mouth open, I close it. Except for that first weekend, when it made sense to have a big strong sit like James, Dan hasn't been at risk for getting out of bed, let alone falling. He had a sit when he first came on this floor, when he was so still that a supposedly experienced neurologist thought he was in a coma. He had a sit when he couldn't do anything for himself except drive the nurses nuts by pushing the call button unnecessarily, and he needs a sit now because he's hurting himself. OK, maybe it's not a sit's job to keep him from bloodying his hand, but it's somebody's job.

After that, I arrive in Dan's room some nights to find that his right hand, the only part of him that he can really move, is tied to the bed rail with strips of gauze. "The early shift did this," the evening nurse says the first time, her gaze averted. "I don't like it. I'll untie him while you're here." She does, and immediately Dan starts slamming his hand against the bed rail. I take it in my own two. "Sweetie, please. Please don't do that. Just hold my hand."

His stare is fierce. No. His stare is angry. He squeezes my hand, over and over again, with a bone-crunching grip. It hurts and I shift my hand, unwilling to be punished for this. I try to squeeze back, but I can't; he has control.

Wednesday, July 17. Fifth chemo treatment—the easy one, through the clavicle shunt—and fifth roommate, Bill—the nicest and most socially adept so far. That is, wearing his hospital pajamas and robe, Bill walks over to Dan and me and introduces himself, as if we might be at a party—a nice party, filled perhaps with academics, men with intelligent, bespectacled faces like his.

"If I can do anything for you, let me know," says Bill, and I thank him, grateful for his effort to go beyond what we are now—me colorless with exhaustion, Dan silent, his face frozen, squeezing my hand, over and over—to what we once might have been.

In contrast, Bill's on his feet all the time, walking around with his wife, a woman with long blonde hair and the lean look of a vegetarian, or visiting with her and friends in the family room. I hear her tell him that the next day she'll take a morning hike with friends who are up from the city for the weekend, and then they'll all come to see him.

I, too, am sustained by friends daily. They drop off roast chicken and Fig Newmans. They ferry me here and there for miles, as I try to take care of the three cars. Yet I'm jealous of Bill and his wife. He can walk, and she has the wherewithal, the physical and mental strength, to have company. They'll cook food together, sit around the table and talk. They'll hold her hands and say, *hang on. You'll beat this. Tomorrow, we'll get up early, take a walk at sunrise.*

After about five days, I arrive in Dan's room to find that Bill's been discharged and a new man occupies the bed by the door.

About two weeks later, I see Bill's wife at the elevator.

"You're back . . . "

"Yes," she says, "he had to come back in."

Her face tells a new story. No more invitations to friends to come up for a weekend. No more morning hikes before afternoon visits to the hospital.

"I'm sorry," I say, and I mean it. I would rather be jealous of her.

I see her again, a few times around the hospital. She doesn't acknowledge me, and I don't press it. If she doesn't want to become part of our community of misfortune, I understand.

I see other people, too, on my walks around the hospital while the nurses turn Dan or change him—Dr. Koerner of the sneer, young Dr. Andrews of the stomach pump—and I'm about to say hello when I realize they don't recognize me.

Only Marge, the sit from neurology, remembers. "You're still here," she says, in the cafeteria one Saturday. Her tone is surprised yet thoughtful, an assessment more than an observation.

Ten days before our scheduled vacation in Provincetown, the owner of the apartment complex calls back. She has filled our July rental and moved our deposit to a week in late September, to an apartment on the bay that she promises is accessible. The Cape is beautiful then, she says. "Many people prefer it."

Finally, I can say to Dan, "Remember our Cape reservation for later this month?"

He makes his sad face.

"I changed it," I say, squeezing his good hand, which is squeezing a hard rubber ball. "To September 24. They gave us another apartment right on the water, with a deck. It's on the first floor." The damned tears start. "I'll drive us all out there."

He doesn't look as if he thinks he will ever go. I don't know if he will, or how I'll take care of him if he does, but I feel a tremendous sense of accomplishment.

"We'll have fun," I say, wiping my eyes, imagining Dan silent, pleased in the passenger seat as we roll out Route 6 toward land's end. "You'll see the Cape again."

Tim Culver, the oncology social worker, calls. "Just want to introduce myself," he says, "I'll help you place Dan after his treatment." He's met Dan, reviewed his chart. Tim's voice exudes kindness and competence. I picture a blond man in his forties, short hair, Van Gogh beard.

"Are you planning to bring him home?" Tim asks.

"—I don't think I could manage his care at home."

"That's all right," he says quickly, sounding relieved. He suggests that I start touring sub-acute care facilities—nursing homes—so that when the time comes, I'll know which one I want for Dan. He's placed people in the Northeast Center for Special Care in Lake Katrine, near Kingston, he says. They do excellent work with brain-injury patients.

"—OK. What about places closer to us?"

He's familiar with Green Manor, which is just north of us. He doesn't know the Adventist Home, which I pass every day on my way to work, or Eden Park, in Hudson, but he'll look into them. "In the meantime," he says, "tour any place you might be interested in."

I go online immediately and find the Northeast Center's Web site. There are plenty of photos, and the place looks like a resort, with buildings tucked in among trees and alongside a pond. Would they really let him live there?

People want me to listen to books on tape in the car, and I know it's a good idea; with the radio as background, all I do is worry, my mind running the same loops hour after hour, about Dan and Dr. Moore, the dogs, the cars, the roof of the house. But the books I want to read aren't on tape. I've been carrying Ann Patchett's *Bel Canto* all summer, stuck on the first five pages; it's not available yet. From Washington, Matt insists he'll send me any taped book I want, so I make an effort and come up with *Girl with a Pearl Earring*, which my mother's been after me to read. It arrives immediately and for ten days—I stretch it out—I'm transported, an hour a day, to a different continent, three hundred years ago, and I am soothed, by Griet's quiet voice as she relates her tale, a life of hardship and beauty. I try ordering on my own after that and get Katherine Graham's autobiography, figuring it will be filled with history and gossip. But I find her insufferable, and you can't browse a tape like you can a book; after a couple of days I send her back and turn on the radio.

What I love in car music is the junk rock 'n' roll we can still get around here, music that Dan, with his indefatigable good taste, couldn't bear. OK, I change the station on the first note of any song by the Beatles, whom I can no longer abide, or "Sloopy," which I knew was stupid even when I was seventeen. But every night I'm rewarded with "I Heard It on the Grapevine" or some lushly tacky song by Neil Diamond or Phil Collins. Sheryl Crow is singing about the communist and his RV. I like her attitude, and I push "scan," looking for her. If I'm lucky, I catch the acoustic "Layla" or the song by Jackson Browne about packing up his piano last.

Days, I try to keep up with the rest of my life. With an eye toward cleaning out the garage, I call a friend who owns a secondhand shop. When Elliot asks me to edit the catalogue for a new graduate program—an important, interesting assignment that I'm lucky to get—I don't say, how in the world do you think I can focus on something like that right now? I say, "Sure."

Dan's always enjoyed hearing funny stories from my office, but seldom this summer do I have a really good one.

"Well," I say, settling down by his bed one evening, "Georgia got back from France today and fired someone."

He makes his eyes big and purses his lips, as in, whooooo.

"Not me," I say. The nurse's aide attaching a fresh fluid IV giggles.

From there the story isn't as good, since Dan never met the graphic designer that Georgia has fired. But I had talked about her. "She was at the container gardening class I took in April," I remind him. "We sat together. We talked about perennials."

Do you remember your first MRI? When I came to work after taking you there, she was sitting on the porch of our office building, smoking a cigarette. How did it go? she asked. OK, I said. There's a problem, but we have some medication, and we'll see the doctor next week.

Does he worry the way he used to? About money, about the house? Does he figure I can handle things? Not likely. Does he even remember the house? Yes. "The electrician came today to move the circuit breaker board the way you wanted him to," I report, and Dan nods. "And I've lined up a handyman to replace the rotted sills upstairs and that support board underneath the gutter on the deck." I stop there. No need to go into my increasingly desperate calls to the incommunicado roofer; success stories only, without the effort behind them.

When I e-mail friends with updates, Sonia writes back that she'll call for more details and I think, *no. That's why I'm e-mailing*. If I'm lucky, she gets the answering machine and leaves a message. But she catches on that I'm home Saturday mornings.

"Bring me up to-date," she says, and I can't snap at her, or she'll report to everyone that poor Deb is losing it.

One Saturday I'm putting laundry into the washing machine with one hand, holding the phone with the other while Sonia sobs, "It was the depression, the damned depression, he loves you, he loves you more than anything," and I have nothing left with which to console her. Another time I'm bringing groceries in from the car when she calls to announce that she will climb the something-or-other peak in Peru in honor of Dan. She's climbed before, in Nepal, after training for months with Dan's daily telephonic encouragement. I tell her that's the perfect thing to do for him, that I'll give him the message when I *visit him* that afternoon. I don't believe it'll happen—I doubt she can do it without him, and I can't replace him.

Often in the evening Dan and I watch TV, whatever his set is tuned to when I come in. Sometimes I ask him if I can look for a movie, but usually I take the luck of the draw—*Frasier*, which has its moments, or a half-hour of Marx Brothers movies. We also see a few nights' worth of *The Amazing Race*, which is perfect for neurologically damaged people—so broad, so obvious, that even if you can't quite hear it, or see it, or comprehend it, you know exactly what's happening.

This life goes on for three weeks or so until the riptide pulls hard again, with Dan usually asleep when I arrive. "Wake up!" says the nurse's aid with the funny twitch. "You got company!"

He doesn't wake up. "Hey," I say softly, "I'm here." I kiss his lips. Some nights now I feel him kiss me back, some nights not.

I put my bags down on a chair by the window and straighten up the room. Whenever the day staff opens something—a fresh IV or a swab for his mouth—they leave the package and its cellophane on his tray table instead of throwing it into the trash can at their feet. This drives me crazy.

"What can their apartments be like?" I say to Margaret.

"A mess," she replies.

I open any new cards that have come in. Sonia sends something weekly, and Lucy from *Time* sends beautiful cards with dull notes—a life in New York without movies, theater, music, or gossip—written in a handwriting that looks like engraving. A graphic designer who has worked on the emergency medical technician series sends witty cards; in one, a row of flowers pops up when you fold it in half. I keep that one taped to the wall all summer, along with a sailing scene sent by another friend, and my own favorite card: a black-and-white photo of a German shepherd balancing four cups and saucers in a stack on its nose.

If Dan's still wearing his glasses, I take them off, clean them, and fold them where the nurse can find them in the morning. I make sure he has a squeeze ball for when he wakes up.

"Do you have to go up every night?" says Georgia one Friday at the office.

"She asked you that?" says Margaret on the phone the next day.

"—She's like that. I reminded her that he can't speak, that I can't just call him up and ask him how he's doing. I told her about the night one of the lenses was missing from his glasses and I looked all over and found it on the floor across from his bed."

Another night there was a puddle of clear liquid under the bed.

"I don't know what that could be," said Beverly, as if I were hallucinating. Beverly is Dan's nurse almost every evening now, a blond, slightly bovine young woman who seems to be taking elocution lessons from Dr. Moore. Half an hour later, Beverly checked in: "Gosh, the catheter must have broken when they changed it."

Another night the room smelled bad, like feces. Beverly shook her head firmly. "We changed Dan and Mr. Sullivan right before you came. They're fine."

So I sat next to my sleeping Dan, and especially when he made slight shifts in his position, the smell wafted over us. I was out at the hall sink, changing the water in a vase of flowers, when I saw Beverly again. "Dan still smells bad."

Only then did she close the curtain around him and then come right back out. "Yup! He's left us a big present."

They changed him then and Beverly came out of the room making a face and spraying everything in sight with the deodorizer they used, a cloyingly sweet, inhuman odor completely unlike him, a smell so sturdy it wafts from my red "Dan" folder months later.

I don't tell Georgia these things. She would tally them as reasons I should have taken Dan to New York, and I would think, but how could I check for his eyeglass lens on a Tuesday night in New York?

I do call Polly, the nurse manager. "All Beverly had to do was take ten seconds to check Dan the first time I mentioned it. If I was wrong, then I was wrong. Instead he spent the evening lying in his shit."

"I'll speak to Beverly today," says Polly. "I've been an oncology nurse for twelve years, she's been one for six months.

"Is there anything else?" she asks.

I hesitate. I could talk for an hour. ". . . urine on the floor . . . eyeglass lens . . . room is always messy . . ."

"Do you want me to assign another nurse for Dan?"

"—The nurses change all the time anyway, it's probably not necessary."

"Beverly's scheduled to be Dan's nurse for the next several weeks."

I freeze. Of course I'd like Dan to have another nurse. But I'm already a troublemaker. They hold such power over us, these nurses. What if Beverly is taken off Dan now and then comes back to him later, because of vacation scheduling. This pause is going on too long.

"It's up to you," I say.

That evening Beverly and I are cordial to each other. But all the cards that I've carefully stood up in two rows along the window ledge so that Dan could see them have been taken down and left in a stack. "Room was messy," says Beverly. "Cluttered."

"He can't see them when they're piled up like that," I say, brushing the day's cellophane and cardboard off the tray table into the trash can. Alone with Dan, I set up one short, neat row of cards.

The next night those cards have been put into a pile. I set them up again. They're beautiful or charming or funny, they're not in anyone's way, and I want them within his line of sight. The staff turns him regularly now, every two hours, in an effort to avoid bedsores. They prop him slightly with pillows so that he doesn't lie flat on his back, and when he faces the window he might see the cards.

The cards are stacked again the next night. I choose about a dozen and add them to the cards already taped on the walls. I use plenty of the hospital tape from a spool left on his bedside bureau, and stack the rest of the cards neatly into the corner of the window ledge so that we can always get to them.

Saturday, July 20. Lulu is stretched out in bed next to Dan with her "a woman of taste can rest anywhere" look. Cooper's automatic anxiety with any new place has finally worn him out and he's curled, a basenji Cheerio, between Dan's feet. We're watching a movie with Steve McQueen and Ali McGraw that isn't very good but still brings to me intimations of life, death, and youth, theirs and ours, even though I can't remember the name of the damned thing.

"I know you know the name of this," I say to Dan, and he nods yes.

"Pauline Kael hated it. She said Ali McGraw's head was bigger than Steve McQueen's."

He nods again, remembering.

"I'll look it up when I get home, and I'll come in here tomorrow knowing it."

His nod says that is exactly what I should do.

On Sunday Paul and I are on the deck in the sun. He's mowed the lawn and dug out more compost (I'm still promising the potted plants that I'll transfer them to the garden). Now he's trying to reset the wireless indoor-outdoor thermometer that Dan's so proud of. The screws that hold the back piece on are the length of an eyelash and almost as thin. While I fetch a cup to put them in Paul drops one screw, and now we're down on our hands and knees, hoping it hasn't slipped between the boards of the deck. Paul is furious with himself, the thermometer, Dan.

"He likes these beautifully designed, complicated, delicate things," he says.

"Tell me about it. I have a Swedish clothes dryer no one around here can fix and a deck table from San Diego that shouldn't be left out in the rain."

We find the screw, but we still can't get the thermometer to work. Cooper scratches at the screen and I let him out. He limps across the deck and falls off it.

"God," says Paul wearily, "can anything else go wrong."

Always literal, I think, *well, yes*, the deck could be more than six inches off the ground. I right Cooper and give him a pat.

But Paul has a way of cutting to the heart of the matter—years ago he dubbed Cooper "Byronesque—dashing but neurotic"—and I can see us through his eyes: it's a summer in which I can't say, *well, things could be worse.*

Dan still isn't speaking. His left side is still paralyzed.

At home, his dog is blind. His kitchen is infested with big black ants and small dumb moths. I've thrown away pounds of food—couscous, quinoa, barley, basmati rice, two kinds of bulgur, grains and pastas I can't even identify that Dan had once been curious about. Now they pour brown mush into him.

When I find mouse droppings in the flatware drawer, I buy Decon and put it down in the basement even though I hate touching it. It works, as always—no more droppings on the butcher block—and eventually, also predictable, something dies in the wall behind the stove, slamming me with the odor of a corpse every time I enter the kitchen.

On the roof, the green tarp that Dan put over the leaking kitchen skylight during the rainy spring is breaking up in the sun. Daily, small squares of green plastic fly away and land in the herb garden or snuggle up against the shrubbery. I have to do something about the roof; whatever happens, Dan will never hop on and off it again, and I'm not about to start. But right now the days are dry, and sun pours in through the skylight.

Defeated by the thermometer, Paul and I pack up the dogs and he follows me to the hospital. But no sooner have the four of us entered the lobby than we're stopped by a security guard: No dogs in the hospital!

I ask to speak with his supervisor and he leads us to a room with a dozen TV monitors. I explain that the doctor put it in the chart, the nurse OK'd it for today, they are *expecting* us.

"Are they therapy dogs?"

"Yes!" *Are we not all therapy dogs?*

"They need to register with security. They need ID cards."

"The doctor—"

"The doctor needs to check with security."

And he won't call the nurse. We retreat, the dogs straining on their leads.

"But they've been here—" says Paul.

"Hush!" Let security operate on a need-to-know basis.

I hurry upstairs to Dan while Paul stays outside the gate with the barbarians, who go into immediate minor meltdown because no one familiar is within sight. Dan's nurse of the day sympathizes but has no confidence that she can turn around security, so I remind her that Dan's chart also says he can leave the floor with family.

"Fine," she says. While she's unhooking him from things and helping him into his shirt and cap, Jane and Judy arrive. They look as doubtful about this adventure as they did years ago when we told them we were going to Nicaragua to pick cotton, but we wheel Dan in his Barcalounger into the elevator, through the lobby, and outdoors.

There are Paul, smoking, and the dogs, whining, all hugely relieved to see us. What there isn't, in this regional tertiary care hospital with 631 beds and scores of families visiting their patients on a summer Sunday afternoon, is any place to sit down outdoors, short of the concrete. We should have a Barcalounger for Jane, too, but we don't, so we stand around while Dan paws the dogs. I expect him to be more responsive to the outdoors—this is a man whose greatest summer joy was a clothing-optional beach on Cape Cod, who dragged me out for a walk under the full moon last January—but he doesn't seem to notice where he is, or take an interest in the sun or the boxed shrubbery or the people. He focuses on the dogs, and then just before Paul has to leave, Dan becomes interested in my daybook. He takes it out of my purse, which he does sometimes when I'm visiting, and turns the pages, staring at each week. My notes are about him—which chemo treatment when, who visited—and which friends I've met for dinner.

Paul and I take the dogs back to the car. Returning to the hospital alone, I see Dan from a distance, and he looks exactly like himself—sitting in the sun, wearing his summer shirt and cap, reading something intently. I stop and let myself just watch him. This is our twenty-sixth summer together. From this distance, it could be any one of them.

Premonitions of summers to come, I hope! his old friend Kate replies from New York.

I hadn't thought of that.

Monday I get an e-mail from Judy.

Albany, July

Hi,

I think we had a nice visit yesterday. I think it was good for Dan to go outside and get some fresh air. I think he looked very comfortable sitting in that chair yesterday. Sometimes he is tilted to the side and looks very awkward. Maybe the fact that they repositioned him before we went outside helped.

I was thinking about the portal that they are considering and I thought of a few questions that you might ask the doctor. Assuming he has his third lumbar treatment this week, will 2 treatments through the brain have any significant effect, or would he get more treatments? If he does have the surgery will the treatments have to be put on hold while he recovers? Also, would the cough he has have any effect on his recovery from surgery?

Judy

Good questions all. I didn't think of them when a young Dr. Somebody from Dr. Ehrlich's office called early Saturday morning, taking me completely by surprise, to interview me prior to my signing another release for a brain portal insertion. I did ask him what the point was, of the portal at this late stage in the treatment. Even a couple of treatments now could be helpful, he said, and also, if additional treatments were needed later, then the portal would be in place.

"—I have to think about it," I said finally, in utter anguish. "That last portal insertion was a disaster. I wouldn't want to put him through that again."

"All right," he said, "think about it." They would be in touch again, he said; someone would call or come by in the hospital.

No one does, that day or ever. Maybe, somewhere, they did have hearts, and in those hearts, they agreed with me. Or maybe they decided his case was hopeless, he would never be a good research subject, or maybe they saw a lawsuit coming. Whatever. They shut up.

The *New Yorker* food issue arrives. He would have read the whole thing the day we got it and told me all about it that night. I add it to the papers in my tote bag. Maybe he'll want me to read something from it.

On Wednesday Dr. Moore comes to Dan's room in the evening, to administer the lumbar chemo. We go over the record review, which has just come in from Memorial Sloan-Kettering. It was faxed to both of us today, July 24, after being dictated by Dr. Symington on July 2, transcribed on July 10, and electronically signed by her on July 17. Then Dr. Symington's office Fed-Ex'd all of Dan's records to the address in New York that I told them we had moved from five years ago. "Don't worry," said a new, kinder voice on the phone when I asked her how they could possibly do anything so stupid. "They'll come back."

Dr. Moore tells me she knows Dr. Symington, and that Dan is getting the same treatment here that he would have received in New York. This ignores Dr. Symington's statement, "It does appear that the patient's neurological condition is largely related to the hemorrhage as opposed to the underlying disease."

Never mind, today's disaster is that Dr. Moore has looked at Dan's midpoint MRI only quickly, and has seen some change, but she can't compare it with AMC's first

MRI. Albany Medical Center sent its only, original MRI to Memorial Sloan-Kettering for the record review, and now we have to wait for Dr. Symington's office to address an envelope correctly.

"I'm so sorry," I say, stricken by the delay I have caused. "I'll call them tomorrow and tell them to send it to you immediately."

"They'll send it," she says, the soul of confidence. "These things happen, you know—in the best of places."

Dan's nurse has time then to assist with the treatment, and I sit in the dark little waiting room by the elevators, jotting down additional questions (has she talked to Dr. Ehrlich's office?). I check once, and Dan's door is still closed. When I look a few minutes later, it's open. Dan is asleep on his side, facing the hall. Dr. Moore and the nurse are nowhere to be seen.

Immediately I make a circuit of the floor, on both sides of the nurse's station, watching for her flowered dress, listening for her distinctive voice. Nothing.

"Is Dr. Moore here?" I ask the floor receptionist.

"No, she's left."

Dammit. I should have hauled a chair from somewhere and plunked down in front of the door. Now I face the weekly sea of five days from Wednesday night to Monday night of no contact, no information.

No. On Thursday I call Dr. Moore's office and leave a message with her assistant, asking that the doctor call me; I have a few more questions.

Dr. Moore doesn't call. A rain shower has momentarily cooled us, and it's dog agility night. I'm so tired that it's tempting to drive the dogs 20 minutes to agility, instead of driving myself an hour to Albany.

I call the floor and speak to Dan's nurse. Her name is vaguely familiar, and her news is good. Yes, she can see Dan and he's ready to go to sleep now, at six o'clock. He sat up in his chair three times during the day and he indicated to her that he would like to watch the Food Channel.

"Mr. Sullivan, his roommate, was a cook at a restaurant," the nurse says, by way of explanation.

Mr. Sullivan is elderly and elfin. He's recovering, slowly, from having his left leg amputated below the knee. In addition to diabetes, he suffers from some dementia.

"He likes to watch the Food Channel," says the nurse. "All the time. I mean, if he wakes up at three o'clock in the morning and it's not on, he gets very upset, so we just leave it on. This afternoon, I noticed that Dan was watching Mr. Sullivan's TV, not his. So I asked him if he wanted to watch the Food Channel on his own TV, and he nodded."

I'm as thrilled as if he had led a demonstration class at the Culinary Institute of America. He wanted something. It was offered to him. He responded. And now the two guys, one in his 50s, the other in his 80s, each neurologically damaged in his own way but still keyed into that vital interest, that life's work, lie in their beds and relive it. The tang of fresh garlic. The heft of the knife in the hand. The palette of peppers and eggplant.

Late Friday afternoon, Margaret reports on their visit to Dan. Owen and Lucy, from Time, were standing at Dan's bedside when she and Steven arrived. "I think they were glad to see us. They didn't seem to know what to do."

"They were probably horrified. They're used to his banter."

"He still banters. The nurse was feeding him the brown mush through the tube, and we joked about slipping a martini in and he licked his lips. It was a really good visit. He was attentive and interested in everything."

How I wish I'd been there. But we're busy at work, and I was glad that Dan had weekday company. Now I'm envious.

"He's always asleep when I'm there."

"He's probably more relaxed with you," says Margaret, but I worry. Years ago he told me that I was a good hospital visitor, calm and undemanding. These days, maybe he'd like me to banter. But I can't.

When I arrive that night, a small box with a golden bow is nestled among the cards, addressed to me from Owen and Lucy. Chocolates! From Jacques Torres Chocolate in Brooklyn. At home I open the package. A dozen. They even smell good. I eat one, and another, but then I stop and put them in the refrigerator to keep them safe from critters. I parcel them out, eating one each night as a reward for getting through the day.

"I'll send you some more," says Owen, and I wish I could hold him to that.

"You saw what shape Dan is in."

"—We'll line up someone for the fall semester. See how it goes after that. The job is his."

"Lauren says Dan will always have work from Brady, whenever he comes back," Sonia tells me in a phone conversation.

"Thanks for keeping in touch with her. Tell her I appreciate her thinking of him."

Lauren is the supervising editor that Dan and Sonia work for at Brady Publishing in New Jersey. Neither Sonia, who hasn't visited in six weeks, nor Lauren, who lives in Princeton, knows what Dan looks like now.

Saturday, July 27. Dr. Moore gave me permission to bring the dogs. I will try to bring the dogs. I call Dan's nurse, get dog clearance, pack up. At the hospital I drive around the parking garage until I find a place near the air but not in the sun, in case the dogs are refused at the door again. I walk them one more time, hating the details of this, stiff with nervousness, forcing myself to focus on my goal. It's another searing day; the tough grass around the parking garage crackles under our feet. The dogs start to pant, and I don't want to give them water. At the walk light I gather them close to me, make them cross at a trot, then move quickly down the sidewalk alongside the hospital entrance, past the smokers in their wheelchairs, the smokers pulling their IVs. "Nice dogs," says a male voice; men always like Cooper. I smile my thanks in his direction and keep walking. I pull the first door open, drag the dogs through, pull the second door, drag them through again and stride to the elevator, looking straight ahead, praying for an open one, which there isn't.

"Sit!" They sit, one on either side of me. I breathe deeply, lower my shoulders. After using these elevators daily for two months, I know almost viscerally their timing. Finally, doors are going to open down at the other end. We start moving first and get on ahead of everyone else.

Upstairs, Dan's in his Barcalounger and Paul's back, dropping by as part of a weekend in the country. "Obviously," he sighs, "the security guards were concerned not about the dogs last week but about the homicidal maniac who was with them."

Paul's brought a photo of Ben, his son, who turned three this month. "You remember Ben . . ."

Dan nods and with his forefinger taps Paul's watch, hard—*tap, tap, tap*—

"Right!" We both grin, as broadly as if Dan's won a quiz show. "He's crazy about your watch, with the light you turn on and off."

I wish Paul would loan us the photo of Ben, but he slips it back into his wallet. He gives us so much, I can't ask for more.

Maybe it's this Saturday—or the Saturday before, or the Saturday after—that when I kiss Dan good-bye in the evening I see him, really see him, as he lies half-sitting in his Barcalounger and I think, *he is not going to get better*. I remember daylight at the window, I remember his looking up at me, silent, with his fixed, frozen expression, I remember pushing the thought aside: *too soon*. Still four treatments to go. Dozens of people are praying for him. We have not given up. The treatment will not cure him, but it could still . . . bring more of him back to us.

This Saturday I reverse the trip, like a film run quickly backwards, driving through downtown Albany with its heartbreaking shafts of evening light on its aged buildings inhabited by people who have the sense to walk slowly in the heat, to sit in the shade and smoke a cigarette, people whose agenda doesn't even include going to the beach, much less buying a house in the country. At home I let the dogs into the yard, take in the laundry, feed the dogs, leave the laundry tumbled into the basket.

I meet Paul, Denise, and Ben at the house they're borrowing, and we go on to the Red Barn for dinner. The owner nods to me as if she recalls my face but can't remember why. I describe the way Dr. Moore slips silently in and out of the hospital and doesn't return my calls.

"Call the patient representative," says Paul.

"I have, three times. She says Dr. Moore is their only

neuro-oncologist. And that she's an excellent doctor."

We help Ben with his hot dog. He doesn't ask about Dan, and I wonder what a three-year-old thinks about people who come and go in his purview, about a man who willingly turns his watch light on and off as many times as you ask, and then disappears.

Back outside, it's another hot, starry night, no promise of rain. We kiss good-by quickly—Ben's on the verge of a restless rage—and they set off north, while I drive south.

And I'm seized with a thought: *So this is what it feels like. This always going home alone—*

No. I am not alone. Dan is in the hospital; the dogs are waiting for me at home.

Yes. I'm as solo as I've ever been. Two hours of warmth and light with friends, then driving home alone in the dark.

All summer, Dan gets flowers. Early on, shops deliver arrangements with cards that say "Get Well Soon!" including a mysterious one signed, "Skip! From Claverack Service Station." Skip must have an application before the zoning board.

People buy something in the hospital gift shop on their way upstairs. Matt and Julie bring a sedum that's still alive today. Depending on my mood, I think that's because it was purchased with love, or because the hospital sells indestructible plants.

But most of the time, friends give him flowers from their gardens. Mike at the office makes an arrangement with fresh herbs that inspires me to use whatever I have. Liz brings gorgeous pink peonies. Maria gathers wildflowers from their field, and Margaret, who's studying for a certificate in floral design from the New York

Botanical Garden, crafts arrangements from the flowers in her garden. In July her day lilies and bee balm draw admiration from people passing in the hall. "Patients come in wheelchairs from other floors to view your flowers," I tell her, in only a slight exaggeration.

Jane and Judy don't bring flowers. Jane dislikes cut flowers—she hates watching them die, she says. For weeks they show up every Sunday empty-handed.

"We don't know what to bring him," Judy says. "He can't eat, he can't read."

"Bring him the Worcester Sunday paper," I say. "Bring the Boston *Globe*. He used to like looking at them at your house. Or bring him that weekly tabloid you have in Worcester, the free one. Or a magazine. If he can't read every word, he can look at the pictures and the ads and see what's going on.

"Take photos of your garden," I say, warming to the subject. "Take photos of the family."

"I don't have a camera," she says.

They bring him a small ivy plant. "Chemotherapy patients aren't supposed to have flowers," Judy says gently, standing against the backdrop of floral color on Dan's windowsill.

"No one here told me that," I say, feeling my spine stiffen. *No. They cannot take this away from him.*

It has to do with his compromised immune system, and germs, and elements that might be accidentally introduced into the room on the stems or blossoms of flowers, particularly on those picked for him by his friends in their gardens. But Dr. Moore never mentions it. Only Beverly, the bovine evening nurse, says something, but she doesn't order the flowers away. I move them a few inches farther from Dan along the windowsill, where he can still see them, and leave it at that.

The ivy is planted in a tiny "brick" building with a shingled roof, a porch that runs alongside it, and a lighthouse next to it. The whole thing measures about six inches wide by four inches high. The ivy sits in the middle of the house, in what would have been a gabled roof.

I can't for the life of me figure out what this is supposed to represent, to them or to Dan, nor do I have any idea how to care for a plant in a container without visible drainage. I try, but it never really dries and after a few weeks it begins to fade. I hate taking it away, sure they'll notice, but I hate leaving a dying plant there, and one weekend when they don't come—Jane's sciatica makes a car trip too painful, and Judy doesn't want to drive alone—I take it home and let it die there.

Eventually Judy does get inspired. She brings in some large, brightly colored magnetic letters and a metal cookie sheet. "I thought if he can't write, he could spell things out," she says.

It's a brilliant idea that we should have thought of a month ago. When I prop the cookie sheet up for him, his good hand moves the letters around crazily, knocking them off into the bed, spelling nothing but gibberish.

"Point to the letters you want and I'll move them," I say, but he won't, he wants to do it himself.

After a few days I stop trying, and then we all start to have fun with the cookie sheet. The alphabet is limited, but several letters can double as others—on its side, the W becomes another E—and we write messages to Dan and each other. One night when he's sleeping I leave him "I LOVE YOU DAN   DEB." When I come in the next evening, he's awake and the cookie sheet reads, I LOVE

YOU DEB DAN."

"Did you get out of bed and change that?" I say, hugging him.

He knows I'm teasing. He raises his chin, lips pursed, as in, *that's for me to know and you to find out.*

On Sunday I face two bills from Albany Medical Center, one from June that I ignored and now one from July that consists of eleven pages, each page attached to the next, resulting in a strip of paper 7 inches wide and 105 inches long. I read this scroll carefully, looking for duplicate entries, services Dan wouldn't have received. Every single thing that's been done to him, every doctor who's ever looked at him, are all here, beginning with Dr. Matthew D. Damon in the Emergency Room. At right are two payment columns, one for insurance, one for patient. His policy has already paid thousands of dollars, leaving AMC to bill Dan for about eight hundred. I pay it with his money, though I know he wouldn't, out of pure obstinacy. But he's having enough trouble staying in the hospital—every week his insurance company insists that the treatments could be done on an outpatient basis, and every week Dr. Moore hangs onto him—without raising the ire of Accounts Receivable.

While I have his checkbook out, I pay two other medical bills. I should probably protest the charge for blood work ordered by Dr. Hahn in May, but I have other battles. And after the insurance payment, Dr. Ehrlich's office is billing Dan $15 for his May appointment. Ehrlich would have had to haul Dan into court to get that $15; to me, it seems exactly what the visit was worth, and I pay it promptly.

Then I do the dog drill—calling, packing, walking.

Lulu knows the route now; when I drive the long curve that takes us off the bypass and into the city, she stands up in her crate and shakes, much as a subway rider might close her book upon coming into her stop. Jane and Judy are already there, giving me their where-have-*you* been look. Dan's in his Barcalounger and completely alert.

"Do you want to take a walk?" I ask him and he nods, so we set off, Dan hanging onto Cooper's leash, me to Lulu's. Judy pushes the Barcalounger, Jane walks alongside. We make a circuit of the floor, push on to another section of the hospital. We could walk farther, but I'm uneasy. I don't want some new nurse to discover our little party and send the dogs away.

"Let's head back," I say, and Judy slowly turns the ocean liner of a chair. At the elevator Dan reaches out the hand with Cooper's leash and thumps the door.

"—Sweetie, it's not a good time to go out. It's going to rain. Maria's coming. Let's wait for her up here." It's criminal of me, but I can't imagine our wending our glacial way through the downstairs lobby, the dogs straining to sniff every single thing they pass. I can't get known as the lady who keeps trying to bring in the dogs.

Maria arrives, her face lighting up as she steps off the elevator. "Hey, Dan, you got your dogs back!"

She's followed a few minutes later by my father and Mary, dressed in much the same Ivy League summer style as the couple we saw in the Emergency Room in May, and looking not unlike them—more robust, but with a refined robustness. We sit in the dark little room by the elevator, placing our chairs around Dan's Barcalounger. Like Jane, Mary seems dubious about allowing beings that use their tongues as toilet paper into the lap of a chemotherapy patient. My father is fascinated, watching Dan, who ignores us, as silent, absorbed with the dogs, he strokes them hard with his clumsy right hand.

"He knew those dogs," my father says for months afterward, in wonder, as if he'd seen a miracle. "He was really glad to see those dogs."

He did. He was. And these days, when I am filled with remorse, when I ask myself if anything I did all summer had any positive effect on his care or his state of mind, I tell myself, *I brought the dogs.*

Monday . . . Tuesday . . . Wednesday . . . Dr. Moore doesn't call, and I can't even catch up with her in the hospital. "She's come and gone," the nurse says cheerfully when I arrive on Monday. On Tuesday, Dan's had his seventh chemo treatment and is tired. I sit next to him and fill out an eight-page application for state disability/workers compensation insurance. The form wants to know how much Dan carried daily, during the course of his work, so I estimate the weight of pens and papers, and note in several different places that as far as his profession goes, his disability is complete.

On Wednesday Dan's asleep. "She was here a minute ago, writing orders," says a nurse at the desk. "She must still be around." So I look, walking to the desk area on the other side of the nurse's station where the doctors do their paperwork, walking by every room on the floor, even the single rooms in back, designated for patients in quarantine, feeling like a player in some bedroom farce gone berserk. I return to the desk, and the nurse is surprised I haven't found her.

"Could you page her, please?"

"She's left the building," says a man in white, without

looking up from the forms he's reviewing.

I will have to call the bitch again tomorrow. I go back to Dan. His nails are so long that I've brought clippers. The nurse's aide with the twitch is changing his fluid IV. "Could someone cut Dan's nails?" I ask her. I say it with a smile, keeping my voice gentle.

"No." Her twitch is part of an emphatic shake of her head. "Not with chemotherapy patients. Get a cut, you risk infection."

"But he cuts his forehead with his long fingernails. Look—" I touch his head near the cuts he makes with his flailing right hand.

Again she shakes her head, hard. "We're not responsible."

"Then I'm responsible," I say, my voice no longer gentle.

"You can ask Dr. Moore."

Right. In silence, while she finishes her work, I open his new cards and stand them up in the front row on the windowsill. As soon as she leaves I get out the nail clippers. I start with his "good" right hand; he's sleeping so deeply that it's finally still. I should be spooked about that, I know, but I tell myself it's just for tonight, just so I can cut his nails. I collect the clippings in a tissue, to eliminate the evidence, and file the nails smooth with an emery board. Then I do the same on his paralyzed hand, where the nails are a full eighth of an inch, since he has no way to tear them on anything.

The toes are trickier. From the foot of his bed I can see the reception desk and, presumably, they can see me. I sit in a chair, a magazine on my lap, and when the receptionist takes her break I spring into action. I get one foot clipped and filed before a nurse takes a phone call. I massage that foot with the French foot cream Cathy brought in

June, waiting nervously for my next opportunity. Having started this, I will finish it. Surely they'll notice, and I'll be in trouble, but I don't care.

It's twelve weeks and two days after his terrible run, and two months since he was admitted to Albany Medical Center. His body is as strong, his muscles as well defined as ever. He understands everything I say to him. When I figure out the damned indoor-outdoor thermometer—"I need to put new batteries in *both* pieces and then reset *both* pieces, don't I"—he nods once, firmly.

And the Steve McQueen movie: "*The Getaway*. 1972." This nod, with one slow blink, equals a smile, agreement and approval.

Albany, August

"I was reviewing Dan's chart this morning—"

It's Tim Culver, the oncology social worker, and I haven't done my nursing home research.

"—and I see that next week is his last chemo treatment—"

He might as well have socked me in the stomach.

"Its only August first. He's supposed to have three more treatments. Two lumbar and one IV. That's three weeks."

"Well, the chart said, 'one more treatment, next week.'"

"I have to talk to Dr. Moore about this. But I can't reach her."

"Yes, see what she says. Maybe there's a mistake." He continues to talk. He's not sure now that the Northeast Center for Special Care is right for Dan . . . more hours of physical therapy daily than he might be able to handle . . . short-term facility . . . Dan would have to move on . . . best not to move him more than necessary.

I bet Dan could handle as much physical therapy as they could give him, but I don't argue. Like Sunnyview, NCSC wants someone they can mend and send. The Kingston location is convenient to my office, but evenings and weekends would mean another long drive.

Home care? I've watched the nurses feed Dan through his stomach tube and told myself I could do that. But what about the rest? How would he get physical therapy? To expect Maria and our friends and neighbors to be responsible for him while I'm at work is unreasonable. Home health aides. We could set up a hospital bed for Dan in the living room. The night aide could take our room downstairs, near Dan, while the dogs and I slept upstairs. I've gone through this sequence a hundred times in my head. If an aide had to cancel, or didn't show up, I'd be scrambling. When the aide did show up . . . it's too close, too many people, too many strangers in the house all the time. I'm surviving these days by knowing that night will bring solitude.

My fury at Dr. Moore keeps intruding on my talk with Tim. "I have to call Dr. Moore now."

"She is a great doctor, though, isn't she?"

I tell Dr. Moore's assistant it is urgent that I speak with the doctor.

"Is it an emergency?"

"—There's been a major change in his treatment, and no one has told me. To me, that's an emergency."

She'll give her the message.

At four o'clock, when I want to leave my office, I call again. "By not calling me, Dr. Moore is creating an emergency. I need you to find her and bring her to the phone."

"I can't do that. I left her your message."

I send a desperate e-mail to Gloria, the patient representative. "Dan and I are stuck with this," I write, "but for future patients it has to change. A patient simply cannot be assigned a doctor that can't be found."

At home I call the hospital floor and ask for Dan's nurse. There's some confusion about Dan's treatment, I say, would she please read it to me from the chart.

Yes, she says, it says he is to receive one more chemo treatment, next week.

Dr. Moore calls at 6 p.m. and lights into me. "Why are you telling people I don't talk to you? I've always been straight with you."

"I left a message a week ago. You never called back."

"I didn't get the message."

"Why not?"

"—I don't know."

"Now there's been a change in Dan's treatment, and you didn't tell me."

"There has been no change in treatment. That order was written in the chart by an intern. It's badly worded."

"I'll say. The nurse on duty tonight interpreted it exactly the same way Tim Culver did. It wasn't just a social worker's mistake."

"Dan is to get three more chemotherapy treatments, two lumbar, one shunt."

I have to believe her. We talk some more about his condition. As usual, she says everything in three different ways, and as usual, I listen hard. Dan's "plateaued out," she says, at least for the moment. She means that his incremental improvements—attentiveness, responsiveness—have not continued. She means that speech, which would have been next, hasn't happened. I ask my week-old questions about the comparison of the MRIs, and she says something vague about improvement. The cranial bleeding looks to be repairing itself.

By the time we get off the phone, it's too late to start up to the hospital or take the dogs to agility. I have to console myself that at least I talked to Dr. Moore. I search, mentally, for what to do with the extra time. The house is dirty and the dining table covered with layers of newspapers and mail, but I get out the ironing board. I've been washing Dan's clothes, but I haven't ironed anything. He has several lightweight, long-sleeved cotton shirts and four pairs of chino pants. He'll wear his own clothes in a nursing home. It feels good to start getting them ready.

On Friday Polly Naylor, the nurse manager, calls me. "I just want to make sure you don't have a problem with Tim," she says.

"—Tim returns my calls, why would I have a problem with Tim?"

"—OK. If you have any other problems at the hospital, Deborah, think of me. Please call. Here's my direct line, and here's my pager number."

When I get to the hospital that night, Dan's awake.

"I'm so happy to see you, sweetie!" We kiss and rub cheeks. His beard is long and full, not trimmed for over two months, and his hair, what's left of it, has grown down the back of his neck.

I don't tell him that I've probably made Dr. Moore our enemy forever. I give him the good news. "She says the cranial bleeding is healing itself."

He has no noticeable reaction to this, so I try something else.

"I have a good office story."

He keeps eye contact, completely attentive.

"Kerry resigned . . ."

Flicker of recognition. He's met Kerry, one of the other editors.

"And she actually had an exit interview with human resources." As Dan knows, this is a first, in the five years I've worked there. "And she said one of the reasons she was leaving was that she had didn't have enough to do."

Inside, he's chuckling.

"Ron from HR followed up on this with Georgia. I know that because Georgia came roaring upstairs to Elliot today—'Do you know what that bitch Kerry told HR! That she didn't have enough to do! How could she say that! I was about to give her freelance work!"

Dan's face is frozen except for his eyes. His movement is limited to his right hand. And now, inside, he's laughing, relishing with me one of my best office stories yet, remembering the dirty little secret of our department, that we editors can sit around with nothing to do while Georgia hands out prime projects to freelancers.

As I leave that night, I tell him the good news. "Bernie's coming tomorrow."

Dan puckers his brow. Bernie lives in Illinois.

"He's in New York visiting his aunt. The one in the nursing home. He'll take the train up in the morning. He'll probably get here around noon."

On my way out, I decide to try one more thing on this hospital, and I stop at the desk. One of the nurses is there, and I ask her, "Is there any service that would trim Dan's beard and hair?"

"Not on the weekend."

"—I didn't say anything about the weekend. I asked, is there a service that would trim Dan's beard and hair. In his room, so that he doesn't have to go somewhere. I know you're busy, so if there is such a service, and if you will give me the telephone number, I'll be happy to call them myself and make an appointment for him."

"The hairdresser makes rounds during the week. I don't know when she'd get to him, but I'll put it in his chart, and the nurse can call her on Monday."

She makes no move to find Dan's chart, so I get out my "to do" list while I have a surface here to write on, and make a note, "Dan haircut," for follow-up on Monday.

On Saturday I turn into Dan's room to find Bernie there. He turns 80 this summer; bespectacled and bald, he's a fresh breath of life in his walking shorts, running shoes, and White Sox cap. Bernie wrote one of the first U.S. history textbooks Dan edited, a prime text in the field. They discovered they'd both gone to Columbia. In the '80s they fell out of touch, but when we bought the house upstate, we discovered Bernie already there, just one town away. They picked up their friendship, adding running to the mix of history, politics, and baseball (Mets—Bernie, Red Sox—Dan). When Bernie moved to Evanston to be closer to his grandchildren, we kept up with him by e-mail and his quarterly visits east to his lively, ancient aunt in a nursing home. The last time we saw Bernie he came up on the train and spent a July night with us. We went out to a revue of Tom Lehrer songs—Bernie's and my idea, to introduce Dan to Lehrer. Dan drove, speeding us through the twilight, as Bernie and I sang "Plagiarize" and "The Old Dope Peddler."

Bernie's brought a big bottle of ginger ale, a Diana Krall tape, and a *Time*, "so you can see what your employer is up to." He makes a good attempt at treating Dan like a normal person, but at lunch in the cafeteria, he asks me if I think Dan recognizes him.

"I'm sure he does. He understands everything that's said to him."

Saying good-bye, Bernie shakes Dan's hand. "Hey, good strong grip." Dan gives another squeeze. "I'll be up to visit auntie again in the fall."

"Dan will be out of here then," I say, "you won't have as far to come."

"Did you recognize Bernie?" I ask, as soon as he leaves.

Dan nods.

"I knew you did. Bernie wasn't sure, so I told him I'd check with you. I'll e-mail him Monday. Want some ginger ale?"

He nods. He still looks jaunty with the white stick at an angle in his lips, but he's not as interested in it today. After a few sucks, he waves it away.

On Sunday Dan is up in his Barcalounger, but he doesn't reach out for the dogs. He doesn't pet them.

"Hey, I've bought the dogs!" I lean over to kiss him.

He looks at me as I speak, then at the dogs, almost without reaction, if anything faintly puzzled, as if I said, hey, I brought the dry cleaning.

I put Lulu on his lap and lay his good hand on her flank, so he can feel her smooth fur and the firm muscle beneath it. Lulu squirms, wanting to lick his fingers, so I move his hand closer to her tongue. We will make our presence known here.

On Monday I get an e-mail from a friend whose 15-year-old son has volunteered at the hospital this summer and got re-acquainted with Dan there.

Luke switched his Albany Med day last week from Tuesday to Friday so he was able to be in Dan's physical therapy session. Luke's unprofessional opinion was that Dan performed much better than the last time he saw him. He said that Dan was able to get up twice on the bars and that his arm strength is amazing. He said that the physical therapists all seem to know and interact with Dan quite comfortably. Luke proudly told the therapists that he knew Dan. He made sure he introduced himself to Dan and spoke to him.

In the evening I get to the hospital early, to put in my bid for Dr. Moore.

"She's on vacation this week," says the nurse. She gives me an odd stare, as if only someone from another planet wouldn't know that.

I have to turn away from her and lean against the high desk. *The bitch.* To talk to me for half an hour on Thursday and not tell me she'd be on vacation Monday, and who would be covering for her.

When I can stand up straight again, I go into Dan's room.

And they've trimmed his beard. "Oh, sweetie, you look so handsome!"

He's awake and alert; he makes his little oohh face, pursing his lips, and I kiss him. He kisses back, long and hard. I kiss his cheeks, his eyes, his forehead—"beautiful, beautiful, you look so handsome."

And he does. My Danny was inside there all the time. "I should have had them do this before Bernie came. He thought you looked like an Old Testament prophet."

He's laughing.

I kiss him again. As always in this hospital, something isn't right— "I asked them to cut your hair, too, why didn't they cut your hair?"

I'll have to follow up about a haircut. For now I love seeing him carved, not unlike a sculpture, out of all that beard.

Tuesday I have an e-mail from our friend Anita, written the night before.

We stopped by to see Dan today after we drove our friend to the airport. We continue to be amazed at how well he looks, considering what he has and what he has been through. We thought he seemed somewhat better coordinated than last time. He seemed pleased to see us and struggled to communicate. He was wearing his white cap!

That evening I realize that without Dr. Moore here, I'd better get on the chemotherapy case. Dan has a new nurse, a stocky young woman with a sweet face. He did not receive the lumbar treatment today, she says. It is scheduled, she reassures me, but she doesn't know when.

Wednesday morning I meet with Glen Waterman, our lawyer. The ballpark figure for a nursing home is $4,000 a month. Dan will go in as a paying patient, and when his funds are exhausted, Medicaid will pay. Because we're not married, my funds will not be tapped. In order to secure the house, since we're joint owners, Glen will write a letter for Dan to sign that states that Dan intends to return home; that way the house will remain in our ownership.

I mention how upset Tim, the social worker, was with me for taking over the one small bank account that Dan and I had held jointly. Glen waves a hand. "You'll sign an affidavit that you put all the money in the account."

"—I did, actually—" but Glen is already onto his next thought. I should liquidate Dan's several small accounts and combine them in a separate checking account for him—his nursing home account.

At the hospital that night, the nice nurse of last night is gone, never to be seen again. A nurse at the desk checks Dan's chart and says no treatment was given.

"Who's covering for Dr. Moore?"

"Dr. Gates."

"Why isn't Dr. Gates giving Dan the scheduled treatment?"

"—You can speak to the doctor on duty. I'll page him."

A few minutes later a young, moon-faced man in bright blue scrubs comes into Dan's room and shyly introduces himself. He seems to know nothing about Dan's case; he says he will make a note in the chart for the doctor to call me tomorrow.

"Yeah, right."

"Someone will call you tomorrow," he says firmly.

The trip to the Green Manor nursing home is exactly twelve minutes, from our door to theirs. The place is less than enticing—bunker-like, one story of brick on a flat, treeless plain. "A little ivy would go a long way here," I say to Lulu.

Indoors is more pleasant, with windows everywhere and plenty of light. And as I step up to the sign-in desk, a small dog greets me. One of those fussy little terrier types, but it is a dog.

A short woman with a cap of black hair shows me around. As soon as she's introduced herself, I say, "We have two dogs that Dan loves. Could they visit him?"

Yes. They would have to be registered as visitors, with their shots up to date, no biting, etc.

Sold.

The home is built in three spokes leading out from the central office area, with a circle of rooms at the end of each spoke housing forty residents. At the center of each circle is a park-type area with trees and shrubs and seating. We could sit outdoors. The rooms are divided not horizontally, the hospital way, but vertically: no more fighting for the window. There are TV hookups. I will buy him a nice new TV.

I ask her who Dan's doctor would be here, and she says, in essence, that's not her department. If Dan becomes a resident here, the staff—medical, social work—will meet to put together a plan of treatment for him. Then they'll meet with me to go over the plan. So I hold my tongue. When she points out that the beds do not have rails, I don't say that the rails on Dan's bed are often up so that he won't fall out of it. She shows me a refrigerator where families can keep special food treats for their residents, and I don't say that Dan eats only the tube mush. All the wheelchair residents I see, no matter how damaged mentally or physically, are in regular wheelchairs. I don't ask if they have any rolling Barcaloungers.

The physical therapy rooms are small, empty, and locked. The physical therapist works three days a week. Without asking I know that you pay for it yourself and it will cost a fortune. I will figure out some way to pay for it.

I'm completely confused now about where we are and she says, yes, it took her a week to learn the layout. It's her first real smile, but I didn't come here looking for friends.

"I'm afraid they won't take him," I say to Tim, reporting on my visit.

"They'll take him," he says. "There are state laws against confining nursing home residents in beds with bars, that's why she showed you the bed . . . they're responsible for coming up with a treatment plan . . ." And, "this is what I've learned about nursing homes," he says. "My mother-in-law is in one. My father-in-law visits her twice a day, every day. And she gets excellent care."

I could do that. Lulu and I could check in early, before work. In the evening I could bring Cooper for his own visit. I imagine spending Thanksgiving with Dan, Christmas. No longer will we automatically be the itinerant relatives. People will have to visit us. New Year's Eve, Lulu will turn 3; she'll sit in Dan's lap. Past December 31, I can't see.

At the office there is no message from the hospital. I give them till 1 p.m., then call Polly, the nurse manager and leave a message on her voice mail. I use the word "urgent."

Polly calls back just before two. She's on her way to a meeting, but she will call Dr. Gates and have him call me. "How long will you be there?"

"I leave at four o'clock so I can visit Dan in the evening."

At four o'clock I'm putting Lulu's leash on her when the phone rings: Dr. Gates. He has a hearty voice, just short of jovial. I imagine a tall man, starting to bald, in a brown suit.

It's OK if Dan doesn't get a treatment this week, he says. Skipping a week won't hurt him.

"—That flies in the face of common sense, Dr. Gates. Do you know Dan? He's desperately ill."

Yes, he knows Dan. He often covers for Dr. Moore when she's not in the hospital. He spoke with her last week and they agreed it would be all right if Dan skipped a week of treatment.

"When did you speak to her?"

Thursday or Friday, he says. He doesn't have it in front of him. He's just come from a conference with another family. He has two hundred patients to oversee.

"That's not reassuring, Dr. Gates."

He laughs heartily, as if I'm a real card. He's on duty this weekend, he says. Maybe we'll finally meet.

Speechless, I gather up Lulu, my purse and tote bag. I am literally biting my lips with rage and terror.

In the car I try to hug Lulu, but she jumps into the back seat: *let's get going!* and she's right: I have to drive home, feed the dogs, drive to the hospital. I have to walk into Dan's room calmly. I will kiss him—forehead, lips, his new trim beard—whether he's awake or asleep. I'll hold his hand and if he's awake, he will squeeze my hand, over and over and over again. If he's asleep, his hand will be motionless. In my heart, I know this continues as a bad sign; in my heart, I know I should want him awake and moving, but when I come into his room and find him still, his frozen stare at peace under his long eyelashes, as if nothing were wrong—for, amazingly, his skin and muscle tone are still perfect—as if the Dan of old, the Dan of a year ago, had just put down his book for a few minutes of shut-eye, I am relieved.

I keep to my routine, swimming mental laps of rage. Others do the analysis.

"Abandonment," mutters my father. "Malpractice."

"He's in the hospital for the purpose of receiving chemotherapy," says Anita. "If he weren't receiving chemotherapy, he wouldn't be in the hospital."

"Someone is lying to you," says Cathy.

Leave it to Judy to ask the logical questions: Does this mean that Dan will stay in the hospital an extra week? Or that he'll get only nine treatments, instead of ten?

There's no one to ask. I will not call Dr. Gates again

just to have him lie to me. I spend my usual hours at the hospital Saturday and Sunday, and I don't see him. I will not page him, because really, I don't want to see him. Dr. Moore will be back on Monday. I practice in my head what I will say to her. In my fantasy life, Dan becomes very, very rich.

On Saturday Dan's temperature is up a couple of degrees. The nurses monitor it, giving him Tylenol.

My brother and Liz arrive, and their presence in the room underscores how much things have changed since their visit six weeks ago. Then we were off balance, but our confusion included some hope. Already today the upswing is over; they've missed it. Dan will take a little ginger ale on a lime-green swab, but he's not particularly interested. Liz can chat to him, but he's not very responsive. It's been weeks since I propped up the newspaper on his bed-tray and read it with him.

On Sunday Dan is officially running a fever, over 100 degrees. The nurse says she doesn't know why—it could be something as simple as a urinary tract infection. Blood work will be done tomorrow, when the lab is open. In the meantime, Tylenol.

Monday evening I stop at the nursing station right away and ask for Dr. Moore. She's still on vacation; she won't be back in the hospital until Wednesday. I can't be more stunned than I already am. It seems Dr. Moore will never return; so what.

The bovine Beverly is back in our scene, however, and she tells me confidently that a urinary tract infection has been discovered. When I ask, she consults Dan's chart and says, no. No chemotherapy is scheduled for this week. He's asleep, but I linger in his room until nine o'clock. When I leave, his temperature is 103 degrees.

Worried, I call the hospital at 6:30 Tuesday morning to check in with the night shift. Dan's nurse is a young man, an unfamiliar voice; I explain my concern and ask what Dan's current temperature is.

"I didn't even know he had a fever."

"Didn't you check his chart when you came on?"

"No one told me anything."

"—I can't be there every shift. I have to count on the staff to talk to each other . . . what's his temperature this morning?"

"Who are you?"

"—I'm his partner of 24 years. I've visited him every day since he was admitted on May 30. We live an hour away, and I often talk to the nurses on the phone."

"One moment please." He goes away for several minutes, then returns. "We can't give out patient conditions over the phone."

"I know what his condition is. I'm asking for his temperature."

"I can't give that out over the phone."

"—Is Polly Naylor in yet?"

"I don't know."

"Will you please find out, come back to the phone, and tell me."

He's gone for a while again. When he comes back he says, "She'll be in at eight."

On my way to work I stop at the Eden Park Nursing Home in Hudson. The social worker takes me around; she's a tall young woman with coils of blond curls to her shoulders, cheerful, almost flighty. Eden Park is old, a three-story building with two-patient rooms, hospital style. It feels overheated and crowded and it's depressing visually, but it has a good reputation in the community for the care the staff gives to residents. Sherry exchanges greetings with people as we walk around. "Visitors are upset sometimes when they see the residents sitting out in the hall," she says in her sweet, feathery voice. "But it's their living room. It's where they do a lot of their socializing."

In the elevator is a poster: an election next week, for co-captains of each floor. That would be me, I think, if I lived here; it would not be Dan.

At this moment, they have a couple of empty beds. One is in a room with a large, cheerfully demented man who's in love with Sherry. He calls to her as we walk down the hall. "I don't think we'll put your husband in with Howard," she says.

The other is a window bed in a room with a man whose curtains are drawn tight around him. Sherry makes no contact with him; she shows me the room, with its third-floor street view, the Catskills a lovely smoky blue in the distance, as if it's empty. "Louis is quiet," she says after we leave, as if this is a good thing.

She asks me more about Dan, and I start to tell her that he's not hail-fellow well met, and my face crumples into a sob.

"Honey, what's wrong—" We're back on the first floor, heading for her office, and she ushers me in, her arm around me, and sits me down with a box of tissues.

"It's not your problem," I say, weeping.

"Don't be silly. Tell me."

"It's just . . . he's so ill . . . and the doctors won't talk to me . . . so hard to get in touch with anyone . . . I'm so tired, and I spend my days making telephone calls."

I'm ironing his clothes at eleven o'clock at night so that he'll have something nice to wear in a nursing home.

Sherry nods, almost in tears, which makes it harder for me to get control of myself, which I have to do. I have to get to work. I have to try to resolve this idiotic situation with the hospital. I have to get the Honda a detail cleaning so that I can sell it. I have to stop by the Social Security Office to drop off a form with Dan's faked signature. I have to thank Sherry for being so kind, and I have to move on.

In the car, I decide to call Ed, our doctor friend. "I don't know how to deal with these people, Ed. They're beyond anything I've ever experienced."

He sighs, thinking. "Maybe the problem is that you're not married and Dan has no Health Care Proxy. Talk to the patient representative."

"I already have, several times. She's been very helpful, but the problem remains . . . any other ideas?"

"The order of things is usually this: you go to the nurse manager, then the patient representative, then an ethics consultation, then the Performance Improvement Board. When you get to those last two, they know you're serious. Ask for an ethics consultation. They'll talk to you, and they can go to Dan's bed and ask him if he wants you as his Health Care Proxy. If he indicates yes, he doesn't need to sign the form."

"How do I find this ethics consultant?"

"It'll be a doctor in the hospital. Ask Polly Naylor to put you in touch."

So I call Polly. I explain about Dr. Moore and her vacation and Dan not getting the treatment and no one telling me. I ask for an ethics consultation and Polly's response is, "What if Dr. Moore called you once a week with an update on Dan?"

"—OK." Once a week leaves me six days without any information, and Dr. Moore won't do it anyway, but I have to come across as cooperative.

"She's here today. I'll talk to her about it."

Polly calls back in the afternoon. She has spoken with Dr. Moore. "She said no," says Polly. "She says you're doing fine, meeting at Dan's bedside."

"That's ridiculous. I haven't met her at Dan's bedside since . . ." I check my calendar. "July twenty-fourth. This is August thirteenth. She didn't tell me she was going on vacation for ten days, she left him in the care of a doctor who didn't give him the scheduled treatment, and she says we're doing fine?"

"—Let's try this," says Polly. "On Monday and Wednesday evenings when you get to the hospital, have Dr. Moore paged. To be sure you talk to her."

"—All right. And you'll have the ethics doctor call me?"

"Yes."

Later, Dr. Moore calls. I'm so astonished I have to pull myself together.

"So, what happened?" I keep my voice low, simply seeking information.

Dr. Gates decided that Dan could safely skip a week of treatment. She learned of this only on her return from vacation.

"Isn't that your decision?" Again, I keep my voice gentle, as if I'm on her side.

"—Yes." And personally, she would never change another doctor's treatment plan, unless it was medically necessary. She'll talk to Dr. Gates about this.

"If I were you, I'd give him hell."

She laughs briefly, as if I've made a joke.

And then we talk about Dan, because really, he is what we have to talk about. He's been receiving the best chemotherapy treatment available for CNS lymphoma, she says, and he has "plateaued out." His fever is not from a urinary tract infection. It may be from the tumor, and she's ordered another round of tests. She ticks them off: a new MRI, a CAT scan, more blood work.

Tests, I think. They assigned him a doctor so that someone could order the tests. And I think, poor Dan. Maybe he was happier when Dr. Moore was on vacation.

No sooner do I arrive in Dan's room that evening than the gloomy Bosnian is ready to take him downstairs for the MRI, so I go along, as he's rolled through the halls on his big special bed. I hold his good hand and he squeezes mine, again and again. His bed barely fits through the door of the anteroom to the imaging room, and there's a delay while the technician sends for help in lifting Dan onto the imaging cot.

"Does he do that reflexively?" she asks, nodding at his hand, squeezing, squeezing.

"—I don't know," I say, and immediately I do know, *yes*. All summer we thought he meant it. Really, he just couldn't stop.

They're ready. I kiss him. "Try to keep your hand still, sweetie, just for the test. I'll wait outside. I'll be here when you're done."

Outside consists of an acre of empty, unlit waiting room. I switch on a floor lamp and settle onto a couch, taking off my sandals and stretching my legs across a low table. Too tired to read, I imagine the room during the day, filled with fifty people, their crying babies, impatient toddlers, adults strained to the snapping point, every one of them worried, some of them terrified. If ever a room needed a night's rest, it's this one.

The technician startles me, appearing out of the gloom, asking for Dan's weight. She slips back into the darkness; her shoes don't even squeak.

Wednesday, August 14. A Dr. Slater has left a message on my voice mail at work. He called after five the previous day, without leaving a number where I could reach him. He says he'll call me back and he does, that afternoon while we're all in a meeting. This time he leaves a number, and I call him right away.

I make a point of telling him what Ed said, to underscore that this isn't just something I dreamed up. "Perhaps you know Dr. Ed Patterson. He teaches an *ethics course* at Albany Medical College, and he's an old friend of Dan's and mine. He suggested that maybe the reason the hospital has not communicated with me is that Dan and I aren't married, and Dan doesn't have a Health Care Proxy."

Dr. Slater's response is just short of derisive. He's talked with Dr. Moore, he says, he's talked to the nurses, and they say communication is fine.

". . . Well, since we're on the phone anyway, do you want to hear my side of the story?"

Oh, he only talked to them first because he was unable to reach me, he says.

"For the equivalent of half a day. I've gone for weeks without being able to reach Dr. Moore. I went for days without Dr. Gates telling me he had changed the treatment plan, and then only when I chased him down."

The lack of treatment that one week didn't affect Dan's

treatment altogether, he says.

"We don't know that, do we?"

If I were the family, he says, I would be satisfied knowing that.

"But you're not the family, are you." He's drowning me, this man, I have only seconds at a time when my head is above water. "And when Dr. Moore was asked if she would call me once a week, she said no. You call that good communication?"

He's been through Dan's chart, he says. He sees that I've signed releases.

"Sure, when they need me, they're all over me. It's when I need them that they evaporate."

Do I want him to speak to Dr. Moore again?

"—No," I say, still gasping mentally. "I'll do what Polly Naylor and I agreed on. I'll page Dr. Moore twice a week, Mondays and Wednesdays, when she's at the hospital."

Why twice a week? Why not once a week?

"Because if I don't page her twice a week, I won't get the information. For example, this new MRI Dan had. If I want to hear the results, I'll have to page her."

Oh, she'll call you about that, he says, if not today then tomorrow, and I almost ask him if he's a betting man. I hold my tongue; don't let him think of me as the wisecracking girlfriend.

What Dr. Slater has decided needs to be done in this situation is that I need to spend more time on it, looking for a Health Care Proxy that Dan started to fill out when he was in the neurology unit so long ago.

Let me know if you find it, he says.

At the hospital that night I figure, what the hell, it's Wednesday, the last chance I'll have to talk with her for five days; I ask the receptionist to page Dr. Moore. The doctor returns the call in a few minutes and I take it standing at the nurse's station.

Dan's had all the tests, she says, but she won't have results before tomorrow. At that time she'll decide how to proceed. She talks about his fever, which is down, and his level of attentiveness, all in great detail, as always. She's apparently chewing something, eating, and I figure she is at home, finally getting to her dinner. She's said a lot of this before but I listen patiently, partly because listening to Dr. Moore is always reassuring, in an odd way, even when she's giving me the worst news, and partly because the receptionist is becoming impatient and I think, *good.* I turn my back on her, the phone at my ear, so I won't have to look at her scowl.

When we're done I sit beside Dan again. He's asleep, perfectly still. I talk to him in my head; beyond greeting him, I can't talk out loud. I probably should, but I have so little to say, and my voice would break. So I hold his hand and think about his day. At about eight o'clock the nurse comes in with an aide; it's time to turn him. Beverly waits until 8:30 because she knows I'll be leaving then, but this is a different nurse, another one new to me. I walk down the hall on Dan's side of the nursing station, this gleaming, antiseptic white world of ours. Several of the beds are empty, and farther from the center, the rooms would get more light. I wish he could be down here, but they probably want him close to the desk. The curtains are still drawn around his bed when I walk by, so I start a tour of the other side of the floor, in back of the nursing station.

And there I see Dr. Moore, sitting, writing, at one of

the low counters where the doctors do their paperwork. And I think, truly, this hospital is the strangest place I have ever been in my life. Evidently, she doesn't wish to see me, and frankly, I'm tired of her, too, exhausted with thinking about her, wondering where she is and if she will call me, weary with her doll-like face in my mind's eye. I walk away from her.

At home that night I spend five minutes looking for the Health Care Proxy, but I don't see it among all the papers in my red Dan file. I don't call Dr. Slater again, and he doesn't call me.

On Thursday Dr. Moore doesn't call about the MRI, and I wish I had bet a nickel with Dr. Slater. Beverly is Dan's nurse again, and she's careful to report every detail of his day: he sat up, his temperature is finally down.

"Did he go to physical therapy?" I ask.

"—Not today," she says. " And he wouldn't go if he had a fever."

"He hasn't gone all week then?"

"I'll check his chart and let you know."

At 8:30 I kiss Dan good-bye—he's been asleep the whole evening.

Beverly is at the desk. "I could look in Dan's chart for you now," she says, "I'm sorry, I've just been so busy all night."

I wouldn't have asked her about it again tonight, but since she's offered, I stand across from her at the counter, with Dan's chart—a hundred pages in a three-ring binder—between us.

He has been discharged from physical therapy, fully a week before.

"Why? A friend of ours was a volunteer there and said

Dan was doing very well, just last week, before he started to run the fever."

She doesn't know, but she'll look here in the chart.

"While you're looking, will you see if there's any report on this last MRI?"

Sure. She starts with today, but it's early yet for the MRI. She won't be on duty tomorrow night, but I should ask the nurse to look again. As for physical therapy, she looks back, day by day, a full couple of weeks. There's nothing but one word: discharged.

"You can call them and ask," she says.

Because we have stood at the desk, because I'm walking down the hallway a half-hour later than usual, I meet Dr. Moore as she arrives on the floor, looking for me.

Can you stay a little longer, she says; it's not a question.

She leads me into a conference room near the nurse's station, a large room filled with a table surrounded by chairs—seating, easily, for twenty. She flips a switch that lights half the room and we sit at one corner of the table.

She has reviewed the new MRI. The tumor has started to grow again. This is a concern, obviously, she says, but in particular because Dan has been given the best chemotherapy treatment available for this kind of tumor, the same treatment he would have received in New York or Boston.

"He hasn't had the treatment now for two weeks."

He had plateaued out before then. Surely I had noticed, his lack of attention, his sleeping a lot.

She doesn't know exactly what to do next. There are two other chemotherapies, and she could try one of them, but they haven't been as effective as this one, so she's not optimistic. It might be time to try radiation, which generally isn't recommended, because while it may shrink the tumor, it causes additional brain damage. We talk for what seems like a long time, without making a decision. I'm to think about which course I want them to take. She'll review the MRI more carefully, and the CAT scan, and come to a recommendation.

"You know," she says suddenly, her doll's eyes on me, "my brother died at forty-two. Dropped dead. Bad things happen."

I stare back. How in the world am I supposed to answer that? What's on my tongue is well, you didn't watch him die, did you, but I will not let her make me rude.

"If you want to see something sad," she says, "go to the pediatric cancer ward."

On Friday I tape FOR SALE signs into the back windows of my sparkling clean Honda and drive it to work.

Polly Naylor calls just before noon. Dan's condition has "changed," she says.

"What does that mean?"

It means they cannot wake him. They came to his room this morning, as always, to bathe him and change his nightgown, and he is not responding to them.

I talk to him in my head as I drive. Hang on, sweetie, I'm coming. We'll take care of you. I'm thinking of you, I'm loving you, hang on . . . I'm on I-90 . . . hang on, hang on, I'm coming.

His eyelids flicker when I kiss his forehead. "Hi sweetie, I'm here. They called me at work, they're worried about you. Oh—" I kiss him again— "I am so happy to be here with you, instead of at work."

But I can't sit with him right now; today, everyone

wants to talk to me. I have to sit in a small, windowless office near the nurse's station to wait for a call from Dr. Moore. The phone doesn't ring, and I'm stuck in this room with no Dan and nothing to look at. I go to the doorway; from here can I see a new, hand-printed sign: DO NOT GIVE OUT PATIENT INFORMATION OVER THE TELEPHONE. Polly is sitting next to it.

"She isn't calling," I say, "can I go sit with Dan?"

"She'll call," says Polly. She puts aside what she's doing and comes into the little room to wait with me. She asks about Dan. What did he do for a living? His skin and muscle tone have stayed so firm, was he athletic? And I'm happy to talk about Dan, how he ran five days a week, wherever he was, and hiked the Grand Canyon by himself, and I'm proud to tell her about his work, the simultaneous massive organization and attention to infinite detail that it required and how he read a Camus novel every summer, and the whole time I'm thinking, why is she asking this now? Why didn't she ask this when he came on the floor two months ago? Wasn't that the time to get to know him?

Polly gives me a little bio of Dr. Moore, and if I'm not grateful, I am curious. Dr. Moore started her professional life as a physical therapist, says Polly. She decided she wanted to go to medical school and from there her path led to neuro-oncology. She's very gifted, says Polly.

Dr. Moore calls. She has a child screaming in the background, and she wants to talk to me. Dan is in the early stages of coma, she says. The only option now, if I agree, is an aggressive course of radiation—every weekday, starting today, for a week. "I just want you guys to get some time together," she says. The time will be short, a matter of weeks or days. I agree because I, too, would like us guys to have some time together. The thought that he might wake up, however briefly, that he might be able to speak, to say hello or good-bye or where's Cooper, is like a miracle held out to me. I sign the form permitting radiation to begin; once again, they haven't called me up here just for my emotional needs.

Almost immediately transport comes for Dan. I walk alongside his bed as we ease into the elevator and then move down a completely foreign hall, into the oldest part of the hospital, with cracked marble floors and heavy wooden doorframes.

The radiologist looks faintly puzzled, as if she's accustomed to patients who participate in their treatment, and the nurse acts as if she'll be seeing us for the next several weeks. I sign another form, and in return the nurse gives me a brochure consisting of dozens of pages and urgings from another world . . . eat your vegetables . . . get enough rest . . . mild exercise.

Soon Dan is wheeled out again and we wait in the hall for transport. He looks peaceful, as if he's just dropped off for a nap in front of the fireplace in winter, the dogs curled on top of him. I tell him this, and when my voice starts to break, I lay my cheek against his forehead. "This booklet says you may develop burns on your scalp, but I don't see any." More than anything I wish I could stretch out alongside him, but the gates are up on both sides of the bed, and I'm afraid to move them.

Back on oncology a young woman doctor, blond hair swept up with a barrette, needs me to sign permission for another CAT scan. She explains the whole thing in great detail before confessing the obvious, that this is the first time she's ever done this. I sign the form and wish her good luck.

It's only four o'clock, which seems incredibly early, here in the hospital on a weekday, and I realize that if I leave now, before the traffic gets heavy, I can take care of the dogs and then come back again this evening to sit with Dan. I kiss him good-bye and tell the nurse where I'll be. I drive home and fuss over my wriggling Lulu, thrilled to see me, and my doddering Cooper, pleased in his own vague way. We walk up the hill in suffocating humidity. I feed them and make my car sandwich.

And then I can't go any farther. I'm so tired, my brain feels fuzzy. I can't imagine driving up there, let alone driving home at nine o'clock. Tomorrow is Saturday. I can go up early. I call the floor, find the nurse, and tell her I won't be in tonight unless she needs me. He's quiet, she says; he hasn't woken up.

On Saturday Dan looks no different, but the nurse tells me he had a seizure overnight—nothing as severe as the one in June, but Dr. Moore has put him on anti-seizure medication. Jane and Judy visit, and while they're there, Dan has several small seizures, signaled by his face, which, usually still, twitches uncontrollably. Jane insists that I find the nurse every time, tell her about every one of them, which works; the nurse calls Dr. Moore, who changes the medication, and when I leave, late in the afternoon, his face is peaceful again.

On Sunday I wake up feeling dreadful, as exhausted as if I hadn't slept, with a splitting headache. Oh no; what if I can't get to the hospital? I skip church, try to rest, creep through my morning routine. I wait till ten o'clock; by then Margaret is likely to be up.

"You're probably dehydrated," she says. "Drink more water."

They visited Dan yesterday evening; his eyelids flickered when they spoke to him; the radio was on, classical music. The room felt peaceful, she says. She brought fresh flowers from their garden.

"I have to start thinking about his funeral," I say, "and I don't know what to do."

That is, Tim Culver has said, twice, that a few hundred dollars can be set aside for Dan's funeral, and Medicaid won't touch it when depleting his funds. I must face the fact that even if Dan hangs on in a coma, he will, one day, die, and some nurse will look at me and ask me what I want to do with him. With excruciating effort, I have put myself into the mind of someone who never said a word about his funeral, even when I brought up mine, and I have come up with two ideas. He loved the Zen Mountain Monastery, across the river in Mt. Tremper. He went on a weekend retreat there years ago and occasionally attended the Sunday service. Every December, when he made his annual donations, he gave them several hundred dollars, as if saying, *I'm here. I'll be back*.

The website of this contemporary Buddhist monastery near Woodstock mentioned a cemetery, but there was no link to it. After circling around the thought for a couple of days, I told myself again that I had to do this. I clutched the phone and dialed.

The voices at the other end of the line were gentle. They didn't put me on hold. They didn't say that they weren't available, they couldn't give me that information, I must call back another time. The woman who answered the telephone told me that I must speak to Sensei Shugen Arnold, and he was right here.

Yes, said Sensei Shugen, Dan can be buried here, as long as it's what he wants. He has to express that wish.

"—All right," I said. I didn't say, this is a man who couldn't face his mortality long enough to designate a Health Care Proxy, and now he can't talk. I said, "I'll talk to him about it."

"I'm not going to worry about Last Rites, or whatever they call it now," I tell Margaret today. "He wouldn't care about that. I could have his remains cremated. Then, his ashes could be buried at the Zen Mountain Monastery—if I tell them that was what he wanted—or, I could take his ashes out to the Cape and rent a boat and scatter him off Long Beach in Truro. Probably he'd like that best, but it's such a long trek out there for anyone to make."

"We'll trek out," says Margaret. "But back up a minute. I know Dan doesn't care about Last Rites or whatever they call it now, but his mother does. I think you should call the chaplain at the hospital and ask that he administer them. It. Dan won't know the difference, it might help him, and it will make his mother feel much better."

In my heart, I'd love Dan to have Last Rites. I held back because I thought he'd be appalled if he knew, and furious, but I agree with Margaret, also a lapsed Catholic, about the potential for Dan's soul and his mother's comfort, and I say OK, I'll call the chaplain Monday.

Feeling better, I decide to take Lulu to the hospital for company. I call for dog clearance, and the nurse hesitates. Dan's room has been changed, to the back row on the floor, private rooms for people with severely compromised immune systems. If I hadn't made this call, I would have turned the corner into his room to find Dan vanished.

To get even, I bring Lulu. She skitters into the hospital and up to the fourth floor, where I can't quite avoid the desk; they see us before I make the sharp turn to the right, toward the back, then another right turn, checking room numbers on the doors . . . and there he is.

They have him propped on his left side, facing the window, which looks out on the Albany city scene, a mix of two-story houses and stores from another era, hanging on in the shadow of the hospital's hulk.

"Hi sweetie." His eyelids flicker, and I kiss his forehead. "It's Lulu and me." I sit down on the bed and put Lulu near his knees. "This is a nice room they moved you to. It has a view of the neighborhood, and it's quiet back here. Peaceful. They seem to have moved all your things. Let me check . . . yes, your hat and shirt are here in the closet, your toilet kit. And they moved Margaret's new flowers—phlox and black-eyed Susans, they're gorgeous, I wish you could see them. Maybe you will, later this week.

"They've put all your cards in two plastic bags here on the windowsill. I'll set them up later, there's a little bulletin board on the wall, and I'll use the sill. Your radio is here by the bed, set to WMHT, I hope you can hear it. I bet you can. And let me check the drawer—yes, your glasses and papers are here. Good. I guess they moved everything.

"Lulu, *sit*. It's Sunday, Dan, and I didn't bring Cooper. It's so hard for him to travel, I thought he'd be happier if we just got out of his hair for a while. If you want to see him next weekend, I'll bring him.

"It's still beastly hot, it was already 75 degrees at 7:30 this morning. I wonder what you would have done, working at home this summer. I fear you would have been miserable. But we would have figured out something. You could have used a carrel at the college library, or one of their big tables with a view of the mountains."

Sam visits, bringing cosmos and coneflowers from his garden, along with Queen Anne's lace, the weed we all love. He kisses Dan's cheek and there's just the slightest flicker in Dan's eyelids. Like Ed and Susan, Sam is an old friend from our Central America Committee days, 15 years ago and more. We talk about his next trip—since the death of his wife four years ago, he's traveled often, and far—Vietnam, Australia, New Zealand. If I understood his impetus before this, and I think I did, I do wholeheartedly now. In my fantasies, Lulu and I drive west in my red Jetta, on a slow, meandering trip that takes weeks and ends only when the Pacific Ocean laps at our toes.

Sam leaves, and the room is ours again. Lulu curls into a tight circle at Dan's feet. I pin some of the brightest cards to the small bulletin board and set up several more on the sill, arranging them in tandem with the flowers and photographs. I get out the cookie sheet and spell out I LOVE YOU DAN—DEB and prop it up where he would be able to see it.

And really, I think that he might. He hasn't had a seizure all afternoon, and I think that the radiation will work, to wake him, even for a couple of days. Lulu and I go out into the blast-furnace world, we ride home in our air-conditioned car to our oven of a house, and I still think that before things get worse, they will get better.

Neil Diamond, one of my guilty pleasures, is giving a concert in Albany in September, in an arena that holds thousands of people, and the oldies station plays a song by him every time I turn it on—"Cherry" or "Brooklyn Roads," or my favorite, the one about the preacher on the hot August night. Really, what I'd like to do is go to a good, tacky Neil Diamond concert. But not by myself, and I can't think of a single friend who would even consider it.

I call Paul and tell him about the Zen Mountain Monastery and Long Beach on Cape Cod. "They're both beautiful ideas, Deb," he says. "Whatever you want."

I call Judy and Jane. I don't talk about the Zen Mountain Monastery and Long Beach. I tell Judy that I'm going to call the Catholic chaplain in the morning, and I ask her if they would like me to try to schedule the ministration to the sick (I've looked it up) when they can be there. Judy checks with Jane and comes back. No, she says, just have the chaplain administer it whenever he can schedule it.

11 p.m.: 81 degrees out, 77 degrees in. If we have a funeral at the Zen Mountain Monastery, people can come up from New York for it, they can come down from Albany and Vermont and the Adirondacks, they can come over from Worcester. And then Dan will be somewhere. I could visit him. I could also separate out some of the ashes and cast them into the sea by myself. I'm happy about these ideas, if a little guilty about the Zen Mountain Monastery. What will I tell them?

Monday I drive Dan's Trek to work with its FOR SALE signs in the windows. Hardly have I sat down when Ed, our doctor friend, calls and asks if I've thought about hospice as part of Dan's care. Sam's wife died in hospice and he must have called Ed the minute he got home from his visit yesterday. Hospice would offer Dan the kind of care he needs now, says Ed. Care that would keep him comfortable, without a lot of intrusive, at this point unnecessary, tests.

Yes, I want Dan to go into hospice when it's time, I tell Ed. But I also want them to finish this course of radiation, and "if Dan wakes up in hospice and has to be moved to a nursing home, and later, back into hospice, it just seems like so much moving around for him. I'd rather move him into a nursing home once, then into hospice once."

"You can do that," says Ed. "Or, Dan could go into hospice in the hospital and then, if his condition improves, he could be in hospice at home. It's flexible, and it's not limited to the two weeks they tell you in the brochure," he says. "Don't worry about that. Just think about it."

"I will," I say, although my mind is made up. Green Manor first. Then hospice.

I call the hospital and ask to speak to the Catholic chaplain. Within an hour I get a call back from a Father Gregory, and I tell him about Daniel, who was raised a Catholic, and his mother, the devout Catholic, and how we would like the ministration to the sick at this time.

"Oh, I can do that only when the patient asks for it," he says. He actually has an Irish brogue. "No, I can't do it just because a mother wants it."

I sigh, defeated again.

"But I can give him a blessing."

My heart lifts. "That would be wonderful, Father. Thank you."

"I'll visit him today."

After lunch Elliot, my supervisor, calls me into his office. His golf tan is perfect at this point in summer, but his brow is creased. He's worried about work. There's a lot of it, he says, and he needs me, with my five years of experience, fully on board.

I listen. This is my job. I need a job, and I'll never find

another like this one around here. I don't say that it's not my fault if we have turnover here like the waitstaff at a fast food restaurant. I don't say that if we're so busy, maybe he shouldn't take off every Wednesday afternoon to play golf. I don't say, I'm not worried about work, I'm worried about keeping my sanity.

In fact, I had been going to ask Elliot this afternoon if someone else could finish up the new graduate program catalogue, confessing that I couldn't focus on such a large project with so many facets. Now I don't. I describe, again, Dan's coma and the radiation treatment and its one-week duration. I say that at the end of this week, Dan will be moved to a new facility, closer to home, and it will be easier for me to visit him. I tell Elliot that I'll take more work home, and I ask him to hang on for another week.

Father Gregory calls. "I visited with Daniel," he says, "and I spoke with him, and I could tell that he wanted the ministration, so I administered it."

"He spoke to you? He's awake?"

"—No, my dear, but I sat with him, and I spoke to him, and I could tell, that if he could speak, he would ask for the ministration."

Next best thing, I guess. "Thank you, Father. . . . Did you bless him, too?"

"I did. We are all blessed, my dear, and now Daniel is specially blessed."

I am smiling into the phone. "Thank you, Father. I believe that too."

When I get to the hospital that night I check in with the nurse at the main desk. There's been no improvement, and Dan vomited during the day, so the tube feeding has been stopped.

"Doesn't he need the nourishment to strengthen him for the radiation treatments?"

It's a question, not an order. I am seeking information.

He could suffocate, she says, and I say yes, I understand that, but . . . would she page Dr. Moore for me, please. Yes, she says. I stand at the desk until she finds Dr. Moore's page number and calls it.

In Dan's room I find Gail and Sandy, standing on the far side of the bed, slightly dumbfounded. All summer they've promised to visit, but Gail got Lyme disease and Sandy works seven days a week. They're our neighbors—Gail to the south, Sandy to the north—two tough, self-reliant women, unafraid of mice or anything else.

Dan is propped toward them, perfectly still. I lay my cheek against his forehead.

"Hi sweetie, it's me."

Eyelid flutter.

"Sandy and Gail are here, did they tell you?"

Eyelid flutter.

"We said hi," says Sandy, "but that didn't happen."

"Maybe he didn't remember your voices. Talk to him some more."

"Hey, Dan, this is some fix," says Sandy. "We should kidnap you outta here, take you back to Snydertown Road."

"End of the week," I say, massaging his shoulder. "I want you to get all the radiation treatments, sweetie, then we're history in this horrible place."

"I miss seeing you walking the dogs," says Gail, touching his other shoulder. "The boys and I want you back too."

Tiny flicker.

They leave soon—Gail's two boys are home alone—and only then I notice fresh wildflowers on the window ledge and a new message on the cookie sheet. WE LOVE YOU DAN—DEB + MARIA.

How I wish I had been here. But surely she knew to speak to him. Surely his eyelids flickered.

Two aides want to turn him. They'll be only a few minutes, they say, I should sit in the tiny white room next to the nurse's substation back here. It's there that I notice cards and a letter tacked onto the wall. *Thank you for your care and concern . . . Your tender care helped all of us. . . .* And even, *To the angels on the fourth floor . . .*

It takes me a full minute to comprehend that these notes are addressed to staff on this floor.

I stay as long as I can, hoping for a call from Dr. Moore. On my way out, I stop by the desk; no, I'm told, I didn't miss a call from Dr. Moore.

It's twilight now when I leave the hospital, dark when I get home. Tonight the melancholy Sufi who works the booth at the parking garage is already counting his receipts. He waves me through without taking my ticket. I drive, confused and sick with worry. Of course I don't want Dan to suffocate, but won't he starve to death without the tube feed?

Tuesday morning there's an envelope on my desk. Inside is a kind card, "thinking of you," signed by half-a-dozen of my coworkers and filled with cash. I'm astonished at this generosity, tremendously moved, almost embarrassed. Not everyone in the office has signed the card, so I thank those who did one by one, when I can catch them alone.

Mike's answer is typical: "No problem. These are hard times, you're buying a lot of extra gas, we all just chipped in for a little something."

Maybe Mike put in a twenty. Maybe Elliot put in a twenty. But it feels like the rest put in $5 apiece, $10 at the most. What I have here is $600. I stash it in the back of my underwear drawer.

At the hospital, Dan's eyelids flutter when my mother and John speak to him. He's making an effort. His left eyelid opens halfway. "Your beautiful eye, sweetie," I tell him, "I can see your beautiful chocolate eye. It's Tuesday and you're halfway through the radiation treatments. Soon you'll be out of here . . . " I never say *you'll come home.*

The tube feeding is still stopped. "He seems to be a little more responsive tonight," I tell the nurse. "Do you think they'll start the tube feeding again tomorrow?" She doesn't know, and I can't page Dr. Moore tonight.

On Wednesday I keep my appointment to tour the Adventist Nursing Home, which is situated halfway between home and work. I don't think Dan will ever live here, but just in case I need it, I want to have been inside it.

The Home is a large complex, nicely landscaped with mature trees. Indoors it's the quietest of the three, with the fewest patients in evidence. The nurse manager is a broad, thoughtful woman with salt-and-pepper hair. She sits across from me at a round table in the empty activity room, and for the first time in my nursing home tours, someone asks me what happened. I begin with the run in May. She takes notes on a legal pad in large, cursive handwriting. How old is Dan? When I tell her, she winces.

"He's thirty years younger than most of our patients," she says. "The state is going to ask me what kind of a program I'll have for him."

"—He's not very active now," I say. We haven't arrived

at the coma part of the story yet, and maybe Dan should live here, where the nurse manager takes an interest in him from the start, but what if they won't accept him?

When the story is over, we take a walk around the floor. I see ancient bedridden women. I see a group of people, men and women in wheelchairs, waiting outside the dining room for the supper that won't start for another half-hour. Bored, I fear, the meal a high point. No one visits them twice a day, every day.

I thank the nurse manager. All the way home, and all the way to the hospital, I think about where Dan should live. I'm starting to see Ed's point. There's no reason to move Dan into a nursing home for a week, only to decide that he's ready for hospice care. He doesn't need any more tests; we know what they'll show. He doesn't need a doctor to decide to give him more tests. He just needs someone to be nice to him.

At the hospital Dan is propped on his left side, facing the twilight, and I sit facing him, my back to the window. Dr. Moore has left the hospital and I don't try to get in touch with her. I am sick of chasing her. She knows the tube feed is stopped, she must approve, she doesn't want to talk to me about it, fuck her. She's worn me down, I know, she's got me where she wants me, but all I want to do is sit with Dan. Only now, in these last five days, has he lost weight and muscle. Tonight he's a sliver of what he once was, a comma curled into the bed.

The receptionist from the main desk on the floor stops at the doorway.

"May I come in?" she asks.

"Of course."

She's a large woman, probably in her early 60s, with curls pulled back from her face and eyeglasses on a chain.

She's been on duty most nights—an amazing number of nights in succession—that I have come to the hospital, but never once has she seemed to recognize me. She never acknowledged me, let alone offered a greeting, and I decided that she must see so many people coming and going during her workday that she didn't remember me.

Now she says that she just stopped by to say hello and see how Mr. Zinkus was doing. We talk about the radiation—only two more treatments are scheduled—and she speaks softly, her voice gentle. Her mother died of cancer, she says; a few years ago, but it seems like only yesterday.

"I'm sorry," I say.

Truly, these people won't stop until they have drained me dry. This person I've never talked to before continues telling me about her mother, a bright, lively woman until the she went into a coma, "and I knew the end was coming, God takes us all, sooner or later, but I wouldn't let them stop her tube feed."

"Of course not."

"Well, it made things more difficult for her. Looking back, I'm sorry. It's the one thing I regret."

"Don't dwell on it. I'm sure you did your best." I'm a Christian. We may find Christ anywhere, I remind myself through mentally gritted teeth. If a person needs me, if she cannot see that I'd simply like to sit here quietly next to my dying loved one, then I must extend myself, stretch myself one inch further, and try not to break.

In another minute she's gone, and I can kiss Dan's forehead and stroke his beard. This woman and her mother, having nothing to do with us, slip completely from my mind until I'm driving home and thinking about her, who had never said a word, kind or otherwise, to me, and I get it: *they sent her to me*. She doesn't care about us, she didn't need comfort from me—my hands grip the steering wheel; if I could pull it out and throw it through the windshield, I would.

And then it's Thursday, August 22, and I'm in the hospital in the evening, meeting with Dr. Moore in the conference room. We take our same seats, she at the end of the table, me to her right. She talks about the radiation, which has made no difference, visible or internal. She reviews the options, which are none—I can tell she finds it senseless even to give the last radiation treatment, tomorrow—and I realize finally that this woman is a doctor, she is here to make people well, and if they don't get well she doesn't know what to do with them. Nothing will happen here unless I speak up. For the first time all summer, I interrupt her.

"I would like Dan moved to hospice. At Columbia Memorial Hospital. In Hudson."

Well, she says, yes, we could do that, as if this is a novel idea, one she had not considered before. She mentions the hospice at St. Peter's, where Albany patients go, and I interrupt her again.

"No. I want him in Hudson, and Columbia Memorial has a very good hospice floor. A friend of ours was there."

Dr. Moore warms to the subject. We'll need a hospital-to-hospital transfer, and she can arrange that. We'll need a local doctor, just to oversee the case, but she's in touch with Dr. Hahn anyway—do I know him? He's in our area.

"Yes," I say. "Perfect."

I drive home in the dark. Am I heartbroken? Yes. I thought the radiation would work. That we would have . . . two weeks. But I had thought the chemotherapy would work. That we would have two years.

Am I relieved? Yes. This is no way for either of us to live. Having Dan in Hudson is as close as possible to having him at home. I see two weeks of long visits, stopping by any time, staying late; stretching out alongside his bed, keeping my hand in his.

Why do I think, again, of two weeks? Because that's what hospice gives you; after that, the rules say, you have to move on. And I figure Dan will take his two weeks.

On Friday a hospice nurse case manager calls me at work. She will meet with Dan and me tomorrow at two o'clock to do the necessary paperwork from the Albany end. The knot in my stomach, the one that's present all the time now, loosens a little. It's happening. I've set us in motion again.

The phone rings again: Tim Culver. Someone's told him. "I'll be away next week," he says, "my only week of vacation all summer."

The knot retightens; my one friend in the place, gone.

Tim promises he'll do everything that he needs to today, before he leaves. He tells me who will be covering for him. He says, "Don't worry, it'll go smoothly."

"Have a good vacation. I'm sure you deserve it."

"Good luck to you and Dan."

And Maria calls, catching me at home in the evening before I leave for the hospital. "How's the radiation going?" she says with her usual optimistic energy.

"—It's not." I'm standing in the kitchen, staring down at the wood grain of the butcher-block counter. "There's been no change. We're moving him to hospice Monday."

"—Oh." A big, round *oh*, like a gulp. "—Do you want me to come down Monday?"

"—That would be wonderful."

Claudia, the hospice nurse case manager, is a quietly cheerful person who radiates health with auburn hair, lipstick, and street clothes of warm summer colors. She is pleased that the whole family can be here on Saturday and carries two more chairs in from the little office so we can all sit around Dan's bed. I'm glad too, that Jane and Judy chose to visit this day, and greatly relieved. Plenty of people have died in this family—of Dan's original nine uncles (four on his mother's side, five on his father's) only two remain—but Dan is probably the family's first hospice patient. Judy can ask her intelligent questions. She and I don't have to try to explain this to Jane. Claudia explains it. The matter of the Health Care Proxy comes up again. The administrator in Claudia wants one. She pauses, her brow creased. She moves on. Every effort will be made to keep Dan comfortable and out of pain. Nurses will make that effort. Dan will not see doctors. He will not be tested. Claudia makes a point of asking Jane directly if she has any questions. Jane shakes her head, no.

Jane and Judy leave soon after our meeting; I sit facing Dan, my back to the window; I can see Claudia, bent over her paperwork at the nurse's substation across the hall. The radio is on, with a cool, clear, minimalist piece like flowing water; the classical station has been doing astonishingly well in its selections this last couple of weeks.

I'm sitting this way, my hand on Dan's shoulder, when Claudia trots back in, her face as bright as her lipstick. "There is a Health Care Proxy!" she says. "It was in Dan's chart!"

I stare at it dumbly. A title page, "Health Care Proxy and Living Will," with "Albany Medical Center" and its logo, opens into a two-page spread. On the left are instructions for filling out the form, which starts on the right and can be detached. Under "Appointment of Agent" Dan's full name has been written in blue ink, with his last name misspelled.

Then confident black ink takes over. Name of Agent: Deborah A. Mayer. Relationship: Life Partner. My phone numbers. The letters "dna" have been noted for "Limitations" and "Termination of Authority."

On the reverse, blue ink returns under "Attestation": "Pt. unable to sign but nodded appropriately to several questions and affirmed that Debby Mayer would be his health care agent" and the date, 8/14. Under "Witnesses' Declaration" Dr. Slater—"Lawrence S. Slater MD" has signed in black and the witness in blue.

"The original shouldn't be in the chart!" says Claudia. "You should have it. I'll make a copy for the chart."

She does that, and I put the original in my red Dan folder. Then I check my calendar. August 14 was the day I talked to Dr. Slater. The day he told me to look for the Health Care Proxy that Dan had started.

I need two telephone conversations with Margaret that night before I get this straight. "He did it just for the hospital," I say.

"Yup," she says

"So Dan's mother couldn't come along and say, 'You ruined my brilliant son, that woman had no right to give permission for those tests, I'm going to sue you for seventeen million dollars.'"

"Exactly," she says. "It's a big, complicated system. It meets its own needs."

On this Saturday night we had tickets for the opera at Glimmerglass: *Dialogues of the Carmelites*, my choice.

We liked it out there, the countryside with its rural vistas even broader than ours, and Cooperstown, with its lake and museums. The B&B where we stayed loved the dogs. I hung onto the tickets, didn't sell them till Wednesday.

Now I settle in our bed, the dogs tucked in on either side of me. Night brings relief, black and soundless.

They said he had been as ever the day before. They bathed him, changed his nightgown, put him into the Barcalounger, and rolled him out into the hall. He sat outside his room, they said, wearing his glasses and his white linen newsboy cap, watching everything with great interest.

Did they say, "Hi Dan!" as they passed, always walking briskly on their way somewhere else. Did they like him? Did he look the fool, sitting in the hallway in his elegant linen cap? It was Thursday. Did he know what day it was or what time, did some part of him look down the hall, thinking maybe it was Saturday, maybe I would come off the elevator and see him sitting up? Or maybe he was waiting for Maria, remembering that Sunday when we were out in the hall and she rounded the corner, radiant.

We didn't come. I came that night, after work. He was asleep, lost to me by then. I kissed him, held his hand. I talked to Beverly, trying to find out why he no longer had physical therapy. I met up with Dr. Moore. Her brother had dropped dead at 42, she said. Bad things happen.

On Sunday Lulu and I arrive at the hospital to find Paul already there. I'm thrilled to see him, acutely aware of how much trouble this must be for him, and unable even to go through the motions of telling him not to come. He's brought a large CD player. Schubert lieder fill the room.

"He was staying with us once and I played these for him," Paul says softly, thinking out loud. "He told me that he liked them. I was surprised."

"He loves Schubert lieder. We have a CD at home. He must have bought it because of you."

Paul and I don't talk much; the music is too beautiful to be a background. My mother and John arrive, requiring introductions, small talk. But in all these years they've never met, and now they like each other. "She's plucky," Paul says later. "The T-shirt, the Madras blazer."

So handsome, my mother says. So . . . *Irish*.

When we're alone again, Paul switches to Randy Newman, but after a few songs he says, softly again, to himself, "No, a little too black." He has to leave soon, so he decides on the overture to *Cosi fan Tutte*. It was never one of Dan's and my favorite operas, but today Mozart is perfect.

After Paul has left I remember about the corneas. Yesterday Claudia said that of all Dan's organs, only his corneas might possibly be donated after his death. Now I ask a nurse I've never seen before, whose English seems uncertain. She checks and returns shortly to say no, it's not possible, because of the cancer. I'd like something more official, but she's probably right. My poor Danny, the one thing he had ever mentioned about his hereafter—donating his organs—is forbidden. At that moment I think, yes, I will have his remains cremated, never mind what Jane thinks. If his body is no good to anyone else, then let it, finally, have some peace.

In the meantime, the music on the radio has become awful—some turgid, banal orchestral thing at once boring and irritating. What else can I play for him? In the top drawer of his bedside stand is the Diana Krall tape that Bernie brought. We never played it; now I put it on. Dan's propped on his right side, facing the door; I sit facing him. Lulu's curled at his feet, ignoring the rule posted on his door: "Visitors are forbidden from sleeping in the patient's bed." Diana Krall opens with "S'wonderful," and softly, I sing along.

"S'wonderful! S'marvelous! You should care, for me."

So many times this year I wasn't sure he cared for me, and he'd always told me I couldn't carry a tune in a bucket, but I sing to him anyway.

"S'awful nice! S'paradise! S'what I love to see!"

He did care, once, and I still adore him, so I sing along until I'm crying too hard.

Sundays a sweet Irishman, probably in his sixties, staffs the booth in the parking garage. He has a wide face and sandy hair and a beautiful brogue, and he's fascinated by the dogs. My favorite parking spot—shady, breezy—is near the kiosk, and he's watched me come and go with Cooper and Lulu. "How're the beeyooteeful dogs," he says. When I stopped bringing Cooper I told him why, and he said, "Sure, they know."

Now I should tell him that we won't be back, and I can't. I am unable to say the words: *Nothing worked. We won't see you again*. Surely he's used to people disappearing. I tell him to have a good week, and he sends me off with a wave.

Hudson

I. W.O.N.T.G.I.V.E.U.P.A.N.D.Y.O.U.S.H.O.U.L.D.N.T. E.I.T.H.E.R.

Monday, August 26. I get up at six, do my exercises, shower, feed the dogs. I watch myself as I move, as if from above—calm, deliberate. Hospice can say what it wants about this being part of the process; the fact is, you are acknowledging that you have given up a certain kind of hope.

You have made a decision, momentous in this day and age, not for life but for death.

Are you scared?

Nope.

I take Lulu with me, without calling first to check in with the nurse; the hell with them.

Dan's lying on his left side, facing the window. I kiss his forehead. His eyelids don't flicker so much as tremble.

"Hi, sweetie. Lulu and me again. It's a sunny, clear day, sixty degrees, and you're going down to Hudson." My voice breaks; I have to whisper. "You're getting out of this hell. Maria's coming soon. We'll visit with you here, then an ambulance will take you to Hudson. We'll follow, and catch up with you there." I never say *hospice*.

I.W.O.N.T.G.I.V.E.U.P.A.N.D.Y.O.U.S.H.O.U.L.D.N.T.E.I.T.H.E.R.

I place Lulu on the bed gently, at his feet. She sniffs the blanket a bit, turns around a full half-a-dozen times—it always drove him crazy—and settles down with a sigh. I sit next to Dan, my hand on his arm. The ambulance is due at 11; I'll wait until 10:30 to move the flowers out to the nurse's station and pack the last of his things: the best cards, the cookie sheet with "I love you" on it, the photo of us, his hat and shirt. I try not to worry about where Maria is; if she misses us, surely she can find her way to Hudson.

Dan begins to make an odd sort of chewing motion with his mouth. It isn't violent or exaggerated, so I wait a while to see if it will stop. It doesn't. Gently, regularly, his lower jaw moves, as if he's chewing. I feel I should tell someone; we'll be here for at least another hour, and what if something's happening?

Two nurses sit at the mini nursing station back here; one of them is Johanna, the nurse from Dan's first few days on oncology in July, whom I haven't seen since. Neither of them looks up at me, so I take Lulu off the bed and we stand on the other side of the counter from them.

"Excuse me," I say. "Is one of you Dan's nurse this morning?'

Johanna nods. She's chewing something. She swallows. "Sorry!"

"He's making an odd motion with his mouth. Could you come and look?"

She follows me back to his bed.

"That," I say. "That chewing motion."

"I don't know," she says, with a shake of her head. "I wasn't here this weekend."

"—I was. I was here all weekend, and he wasn't doing that. It's new."

She lifts her shoulders, not uncaring exactly, but unwilling to press on. I could demand that she call the doctor on duty, but I don't. It's too perfect. After three months in this hospital as a man without a country, he is now a man without a continent, no longer even their patient.

Maria arrives at exactly 11—"Hey, Dan, soon you're outta here"—and the ambulance crew 10 minutes later. We stand in the hall while the two polite, uniformed men close the door and transfer Dan to a travel stretcher. Johanna has the discharge papers ready; in a burst of administrative fervor, Dr. Moore has dictated her required chronology and got someone to transcribe it, on deadline. I sign the papers, agreeing that Dan has not been forced to leave the hospital before he is ready, and put my copies into my red Dan folder. I don't thank the two nurses; they don't wish us well. The ambulance men wheel Dan out of the room, and he faces us, the head of the stretcher slightly elevated.

What I want to do is to put his white linen hat onto his head. I left it here overnight so that he could wear it home, if it felt right. Now I'm not sure. He never went outdoors without wearing some kind of a hat. But I fear making him look clownish. Gone is the Dan apparently born with an innate sense of style, reflected in every single thing he wore, from his running shorts to his tuxedo. Today the hat might look like a joke, and this trip is necessary, it's a relief and it's the right move, but it is not a joke.

The chewing is seizure activity, says Jenny, the hospice nurse manager at Columbia Memorial Hospital. But

Dan has made the trip well, she says, without any additional stress. Jenny is slim and muscular, a runner; we recognize each other from local foot races. She apologizes for Dan's room, which is tiny—the three of us can barely fit around his bed—and says she may be able to move him to a larger room soon. There's no closet—this entire room was once a closet—but I hang Dan's toilet kit on the bathroom doorknob, in case there's anything in it the nurses would want, and I check out the small window at the foot of his bed. Half of it is cloudy glass, but it does let in some light.

And here in hospice each patient is loaned a radio with a CD player. Jenny needs to examine Dan now, so Maria and I go home to get some CDs.

While I walk the dogs Maria makes us turkey sandwiches. When I come back I see that she's used a knife from the drawer that I never cleaned the mouse turds out of, and I think, once probably won't kill us. We eat at the green table on the deck, the dogs stretched around us in the sun. She calls Jon and leaves a message with an update ("I love you," she says, signing off), and I choose CDs from the pile that I brought home from Albany in June and left untouched—*A Little Night Music, 18 Inches of Rain*, the Bach suites.

At the hospital, Jenny reports on her examination. Dan has a tiny bedsore on his back—"it's a curve, like the white of my thumbnail," she says, showing me. They will monitor that. He has thrush in his mouth, a fungus disease common in cancer patients; they will treat that. I feel like I have rescued him from Albany Medical Center.

Maria kisses Dan's forehead—"back soon, Dan"—hugs me hard, and starts her long drive home.

I sit next to Dan and fill out a form that Jenny needs. Part of it directs me to confirm with my signature that Dan can stay in the hospital hospice for only two weeks. After that he has to move on, to home or another facility.

"I don't like that form," says Jenny, "but I have to give it to you. As far as I'm concerned, you don't have to sign it, if you're not comfortable with it."

Finally, some advice from a human being. I don't sign the form.

At 4:30 I meet with Glen Waterman, our lawyer, in his office, only a few blocks from the hospital. We sit in the big wood-paneled meeting room. He expresses his regrets that things have gone so badly for Dan. But in case Dan lingers in a coma, he says, I should continue to dissolve his small accounts and set up one checking account for him, for his care. Only now does Ted say the actual words: once Dan dies, the power of attorney is dissolved.

I go home and look at the bills that have come in. One each for our two telephone lines; I'll pay those myself. There are also two medical bills, dating from when Dan was in Kingston Hospital in June, which have only recently arrived—one for radiology and one for Dr. Singh, who discharged him in worse condition than when he went in—and a bill for insurance for the three cars that isn't due for a couple of weeks yet. I get out Dan's checkbook and, gritting my teeth, pay the medical bills. I hate paying Dr. Singh, and Dan would tear up the bill, but the last thing I need is a skip tracer at the door.

Then I stare at the car insurance bill, which I need to pay with his money. A quarterly payment would be fairest to him, using the least of his money. I have two of the cars for sale; within weeks they may not need to be insured.

But what if I don't have enough money, after he dies? The semiannual payment would be a good compromise.

But how nice it would be, not to have to worry about this one thing, for a whole year.

"Sweetie," I say, "you have to do this for me," and feeling like a character in *Double Indemnity*, I pay the whole bill, $1,262, with his money, and mail the checks that evening on my way into the hospital.

On Tuesday at 8 a.m. two HVAC technicians begin their day's work of installing a new heating oil tank and hot-water heater at our house. I settle at the kitchen table with a project from my office. Jenny calls mid morning to say they have moved Dan to a larger, nicer room. It takes her a long time to tell me this, as if she's underscoring their thoughtfulness. Irene, the hospice counselor, would like to meet with me this afternoon, says Jenny, is that possible? Sure, I say. I had planned to go to the office in the afternoon, but I'd much rather go to the hospital.

Dan's room is now at the other end of the hall, the farthest from Jenny's office and the nursing station, a big corner room with a small window looking out over the city and beyond it, the Catskills. The window is across the room from the foot of the bed; if he were awake, he wouldn't be able to see anything out of it but the sky, but he's not awake, so the room, with its larger space and brighter light, is an improvement. Next to the window is a small bulletin board; I select the absolute best half-dozen of his cards and pin them up. I talk to Dan as I work, telling him which cards I'm using (the pop-up flowers, the German shepherd with the cups and saucers, a new wacky one from Lucy at *Time* that features Queen Elizabeth) and why. I describe his view to him and tell him about the installation, how the two men drained our old heating oil tank, then carried it up the cellar stairway in pieces.

Then I sit down next to him and discover that this room comes with a crummy radio. It doesn't play CDs and it's stuck on a local talk station that would have driven him nuts. Radio in hand, I walk down the hall. A comatose patient lies in Dan's previous bed, alone in the little room with the half window; on the sill is the other radio. I pause at the door, wishing for help, knowing I shouldn't go into another patient's room, especially when he can't defend his radio. When I see a nurse nearby I ask her if I might please exchange the radios.

"They're all the same," she says with a shrug.

"No, they're not. This one doesn't play CDs, and it's stuck on a station he hates."

She examines the radio to confirm these accusations before she gives me the other one. I walk back down the hall with it cradled in my arm and put on the Bach cello suites.

Irene is not able to meet with me after all—she has to deal an emergency at the hospice unit across the river—and Jenny acts as if they have inconvenienced me terribly while I keep telling her it doesn't matter, this is where I want to be. Still, I leave at four to tip the HVAC team. The leader, with a smudge of oil on his forehead, proudly shows me our new home heating oil tank, which is indeed beautiful and a great relief over the corroded one.

"This is primer," he says, tapping its shiny gray surface. "You could leave it like this, but to protect your investment, you should give it a coat of Rustoleum."

"—OK . . ." I try to nod as if I know what he's talking about.

"—You go to Wal-Mart," he says, catching on. "Buy a pint—no more—of Rustoleum, a roller, a brush, and a pan. That's all you need. You roll the sides and brush the ends."

"OK," I say, with another, more confident, nod. In my mind's eye I see myself spattered with oil-based black paint; just possibly, I might be able to do this project.

At the hospital that evening, Dan's temperature is 102 and he's having facial seizures again, not the little chewing ones but the larger ones, in which his whole face moves. The nurse has a call into Dr. Hahn, who eventually responds, permitting Tylenol and prescribing a mild anti-seizure medication.

Dan's also had diarrhea while I was home; they've cleaned him up, and a large plastic hamper in the room is filled with bedding that doesn't smell good. Presumably it can't go to the laundry until morning, so I roll it into a corner, as far from the bed as possible. Then I put on Bach again and try to do some work, but it's impossible; the work I do is too stupid to be done in this room.

On Wednesday, August 28, I go to the hospital first thing. Dan is as ever, yet quieter; his eyelids no longer even tremble when I speak to him. In a room near his, a woman cries out. "No, no, *no*," she wails; her voice is young and strong, her anguish palpable. I'd like to close our door a little, but the room already smells, from the laundry hamper, which is exactly where I left it last night. In the hallway, other patients' hampers stand to the left of their doors, waiting for the Bangladeshi women who work in the laundry to come by for them. I push Dan's hamper out of his door, and from nowhere a well-dressed woman materializes and says I can't do that.

"Everyone else's is out," I say.

"There's a risk of contamination here," she says.

"It's been in his room since last night. It smells terrible."

"No." She shakes her head. "Those are from this morning."

"They're smelling up the whole room."

"I'll get someone to take them right away," she says, and charges off down the hall. I sit next to Dan, staring at the sheets in the clear plastic hamper, which are in exactly the same configuration as they were last night.

In a few minutes, the woman is back. "There's no one available," she says, "I'll take them myself," and in her summer suit, her gold necklace and bangle bracelets, she rolls the hamper.

"Thank you, I would have done that."

"It's all right," she says. "I apologize for the delay."

Immediately the room smells fine. "Weird morning here," I say to Dan.

At nine Jenny comes in and says Irene will absolutely see me at two o'clock this afternoon, so I go home and try to work there. At noon I go back to the hospital and find our friend Cathy sitting by Dan, reading to him from the food section of the New York *Times*. She has taken the train up from New York and walked from the station.

"I asked the station master for directions," she says, "and he said it was a very long walk, I should take a taxi. But I wanted to walk, so I bought a bottle of water for the trek, and then I was here in ten minutes."

We go to a diner nearby for lunch, and when we get back, Dan's breathing is labored and I lose more time with him while I look for Jenny to tell her this. Then Cathy gets to sit with Dan—"I'll read him the restaurant review"—while I meet with Irene in what's called the family room, a large room with a table and chairs, refrigerator, couches, all brightened by a wall of windows looking out on the mountains.

Irene is a friendly, no-nonsense type in her fifties with the leathery tan of a golfer. Alone in the room, we take chairs at the table. She apologizes for missing our meeting yesterday, for the woman wailing and the smelly laundry. Jenny comes in to inform us that she would like to give Dan a shot of morphine to ease his breathing. This is a common solution, she explains, and I agree to it. Then Irene talks to Jenny about the laundry and the woman wailing and I say never mind, this is a hospital, after all, and Jenny says she really would like to get back to Dan to give him this shot. She leaves, and Irene turns to me.

"You're probably wondering why this happened to you," she says.

And I know she means well, but I am weary, after a summer of being brave and polite and understanding, and I say, "No, I'm not . . . Do you know Dr. Patterson?"

She nods; everyone around here knows Ed.

"When his son died at nine, in a house fire, I learned that none of us is safe from tragedy. A year later, a friend's three-year-old daughter died of a virus, in a New York hospital, after the best care that money could buy. Being middle class and educated mean nothing.

"Dan and I have lost four friends to cancer, three of them in the last four years. Three of them were in their forties; the other one was in his fifties, just a year older than we were."

When I was in my twenties, a friend's son and brother, flying in a small plane, were killed when it crashed. My friend lost his only son, his only brother. In high school, a boy in my class drowned in a swimming accident. Another boy, from church, died in a car accident. No drugs, no alcohol; simply tragic accidents, my first funerals. I can still see the faces of their mothers. One could keep her chin up. The other had to be helped from the church.

I don't tell her these last—she'll think I'm obsessed with death—but they are always part of my backstory.

"I feel many things, Irene, but I don't feel singled out."

When Cathy leaves, I walk downstairs with her and go to the bank right before it closes. I need my signature witnessed for my written request to close Dan's Dreyfus account. In my purse is the check from the close-out of his Prudential Bache account, and I know I should set up the new separate checking account for Dan or at least deposit the check in my account but I can't decide which to do (Glen would veto the latter) and it will take time and I want to get back to Dan. I promise myself I will set up the account tomorrow morning.

Dan's nurse that evening is a small woman with a pageboy of graying brown hair, who introduces herself crisply as Mrs. Armitage. In the last one hundred days I must have met a hundred nurses, every single one of whom has referred to him- or herself by first name: Gwen, Brad, Beverly, Johanna. And tonight we draw this little soldier who refers to herself as Mrs. Armitage. Fighting off what must be mild hysteria—she reminds me of something in *Young Frankenstein*—I return the introduction. "I'm Deborah. This is Daniel," my palm resting on his shoulder.

I've brought my sandwich dinner, planning to eat it at a table, civilized. Dan is quiet. "It's six-thirty," I tell him.

"Evening. I'm going to eat a sandwich in the family room. It's just down the hall. *A Little Night Music* still has a ways to go." He loves that show. We've seen it three times; whenever summer stock did it, we were there.

In the family room three men sit at one end of the table, eating, chatting; they don't acknowledge me. I unpack my sandwich, V-8 juice, my paper napkin and straw. I miss my iced coffee, but in the refrigerator are small cans of generic soda; something to look forward to later.

As I eat, the sun begins to set, and it's a sherbet sunset over the liquid blue-gray of the mountains, one of the lushest sunsets I've ever seen in my life, swaths of raspberry and orange, drifts of white clouds, an edible sunset like the Creamsicles of my childhood. Dan and I have seen gorgeous sunsets in Costa Rica and Mexico, we've watched the sun set in Marin County and from our rooftop in Manhattan, but I have never seen anything like this . . . *aggressive* sunset. I get up and sit against the couch back so that I'm closer to the window, with nothing before me but the sunset. Behind me the men continue to eat and chat; they must come here every night. I should go back to Dan . . . how he would love this . . . we would have held hands, watched it like a movie . . . maybe we can see part of it from his room. Still, I'm unable to budge—I'll never see anything like this again—until finally the colors fade just a bit.

A Little Night Music has ended. "There's the most beautiful sunset . . ." but Dan's small window faces southwest, offering just tendrils of pink, and besides, his breathing seems labored again. I sit down next to him for a minute, my hand on his shoulder, and I decide yes: "I'm going to find the nurse—I'll be right back."

I walk down the hall and stop at the nursing station without seeing Mrs. Armitage or anyone else. I continue toward Dan's old room, and Mrs. Armitage comes out of it. I tell her the problem, and what Jenny did this afternoon, and she says she will be right there. She doesn't follow me to Dan's room, so I sit down next to him again and look at my watch. "I'll give her five minutes," I tell him.

In four minutes Mrs. Armitage appears, looks at Dan, nods, and says she'll be right back. In another four minutes she's back with a needle and gives him a shot.

"There," I tell him, "that should help soon."

It's about 7:30. I put on *Eighteen Inches of Rain* by Ian Tyson and take off my sneakers so I can stretch my legs up onto his bed. I lean against his mattress and keep my hand on his warm forearm, smooth with its fine black hairs.

At eight o'clock his breathing hasn't changed and I'm wondering how long this is supposed to take, when Ed Patterson calls. Visiting the hospice floor on rounds today, he discovered Dan there. I describe Dan's breathing and the morphine shots. "But it hasn't worked yet."

"It can take a little while," he says, reassuring, "as much as an hour."

"That was Ed, sweetie. The medicine should start to work soon."

At 8:30 Dan's breathing is no better, and I'm glad I don't have to leave. I wish someone would come in to check on us, but the hallway is empty. When I'm not stretched alongside Dan's bed, my feet next to the curve that represents his legs, I stand, watching him breathe, amazed at his strength. His chest heaves largely, rhythmically as he breathes in and out through his mouth, as if he were doing an exercise. His eyes are closed; he's doing nothing but breathing, his whole body a pump—a big, strong pump. His brain has shut down, I tell myself, only his body is working; he has no fear, no sense of choking. I've read this somewhere; I pray that it's true.

And then, around nine o'clock, it gets worse. He goes from breathing to gasping for breath. I look out in the hall; no one there. I go back to the bed, afraid to leave him. He is gasping. We need help. My sneakers are off. I put one on, tie it; he is gasping. I put the other on, don't tie it, hop down the hall. I must do this very, very quickly. There are three nurses in the station, none of whom is Mrs. Armitage. They are talking to each other and don't look at me.

"Excuse me—please, I need help. Dan's breathing is very bad."

"Dad?" says one of them vaguely, a tall blond one I've seen before.

"Dan! Dan Zinkus! Please! We need help now!"

She's made eye contact; she's stuck following me. I hop back down the hall.

He hasn't changed, he's still gasping. "See, this is what I mean—"

I can feel her standing at my left, slightly behind me. "He's breathing his last," she says, surprised yet sure.

"—He is?"

She puts her arm around me and kisses my cheek. I want to pull away, but I don't; she's all I have, and she has seen this before.

We stand there, my hand on Dan's arm, the only steady part of him as his chest heaves, rising off the bed and lowering again. I don't tell him not to go, there's no telling him not to go. I say, "We're here, sweetie. We're here." *You aren't alone.* And in another couple of minutes he stops gasping, and his left eyelid slides up half way.

"Oh, sweetie, I can see your eye again, your beautiful chocolate eye."

Just because you're on the hospice floor in this hospital doesn't mean you have a hospice nurse. I sit with my palm curved over Dan's smooth, warm forehead while the tall blond nurse fetches Mrs. Armitage, who says that she will contact the hospice nurse who's on call tonight. She returns to say that nurse is on her way over from the other side of the river . . . would I like tea, or a soda? I was going to drink one of those little cans of soda, I say, and she brings me one, intriguing in its smallness, with a straw and a napkin. I hold it in my left hand, my right hand on Dan's forehead. The cool, sweet soda revives me. I should call people, especially our parents, but I put it off; I just want to sit with him.

I'm in no hurry to leave, I'll sit here all night, if necessary—except for the dogs. It's 9:30, too late to ask anyone I know to go out, except possibly Chris and Robin, friends from church who have kept me supplied in roast chicken and Fig Newmans this summer. Chris answers the phone promptly, to my great relief.

"Do you want us to come over?"

"—No, thanks, I'm all right, but—could you let the dogs out?"

"There, sweetie, the dogs are taken care of." I settle back down next to him, my hand cupped over his forehead.

The hospice nurse is Barbara, a sturdy, middle-aged woman with brown hair in a single braid down to her waist, and large eyeglasses. She has an odd brogue mixed with a city accent, and a quiet energy. First, she stands next to Dan's bed. After observing him in silence, for a minute, she declares that he looks peaceful.

"He died a peaceful death," she says. "I'm not just sayin' that. I've seen them when they haven't."

To me, Dan looks only dead; he no longer appears to be sleeping, as he did in the coma, and he was unconscious when he died, so I don't understand how he could feel peaceful or otherwise, but if she knows something here that I don't, I will accept it.

Barbara's work is a mix of official and spiritual. She brings me a long list of local funeral homes that I must choose from, now. There is no leaving his body in the hospital while I interview morticians.

"I have to take his things with me tonight?"

"Yes, dear, you should take whatever belongs to him."

And she offers me a prayer, if I would like, and I say yes, and she brings me a photocopy. It's an ecumenical prayer, not one that Dan or I would have said, but I read it slowly and then put it in my red Dan folder. It doesn't occur to me to call a priest or the rector from my church; only Dan's body stopped tonight. His mind went out ten days ago, he's been gone from me for most of this month, and really, he began slipping away from us early this year. I'd rather just sit with him, my hand on his forehead, with this nice nurse coming in and out, reassuring me with her funny nurse knowledge—"I hear he had diarrhea yesterday, he's all cleaned out," she says, in a tone content, pleased for him.

"Would you like me to make some calls for you?" she asks another time.

"—Thank you—I can call people tomorrow . . ."

"Are you sure? I can do it, you know."

It's a tempting offer. Judy will still be up; so will my mother. They might be hurt if they didn't hear until tomorrow. My father will be asleep, and being a more reasonable person, can wait until daylight. Barbara takes the telephone numbers. I tell her that Judy will answer the phone, that Jane is hard of hearing, and I say, "You will explain to them that I just want to sit with Dan? That I'll talk to them tomorrow?"

"I've done this many times, dear."

Yet even a person of Barbara's experience is jarred by Judy. "I guess she was shocked," Barbara says, puzzled, and I can only imagine the coldness she must have felt over the phone. Then Barbara called my mother, who, in contrast, was so happy that someone had thought of her, so warm and interested in any detail that Barbara could provide—for months afterward, my mother will tell me how peacefully Dan died—that Barbara was sustained enough to call Judy again to see if everything was all right. Apparently that conversation went a little better. Judy had made a decision, had waked Jane and told her; the worst was over.

Barbara has called the funeral home I have chosen; they will send someone for Dan's body.

"I'll stay with him until then, see him out when they leave with him."

"—You don't want to do that," Barbara says, gently, yet with emphasis, shaking her head. "No one is ever happy when they do that," she says firmly.

"—I'll stay until they come then?"

She nods. "That would be the thing to do."

I take down the cards I pinned to the bulletin board yesterday, collect our CDs. Weeping, I put them into my bag, along with the two photos—Dan and me, Dan and Cooper—and his white linen cap and cream short-sleeved shirt, which I had hung in the little metal closet so that he would have something there. I sit back down next to him. His forehead is just the slightest bit cool.

Two young men stop at the door. They've been called out from home this evening, and they've put on Navy blue blazers over their polo shirts.

"You've come for him?" I say, and they nod. "Give me just another minute."

They withdraw.

"Well, sweetie, this is it." Tears stream from my eyes. "Two men from the funeral home are here. They're going to take you now . . . I won't see you again." I kiss his forehead. There is nothing more to say. He knows everything. I shoulder my bags, kiss him once more, and leave.

At home, I'm not alone. Chris and Robin are still there because they haven't been able to get Lulu back into her crate.

"We tried biscuits—" And Chris, who is short and slender, stuck her own head and shoulders into the crate, as an example.

"I'm so sorry, I forgot to tell you that it didn't matter, you could just leave her."

I turn up lights in the house, and we sit in the living room. The dogs, delighted with company, join us, Lulu on my lap, Cooper on the couch next to Chris. They let me talk, about Dan, about my plans.

"A roofer?" says Robin. "We know a good roofer." She writes down his name and number.

"Why don't I make some calls for you," she says, her notebook still out. I hesitate, then give her Elliot's number at work, and Mike's. I can hear Robin's voice tomorrow morning, at exactly 9 a.m., warm, yet professional. This becomes a good idea, and I give her other names and numbers as we sit.

"Will you be all right?" they say, and I say, "yes, I've been alone since May 30, it'll be the same, only different," and it's Robin who voices it, *the transition's been going on all summer*.

Still, I feel lucky they were here, freshly solitary when they leave. I watch myself put Lulu into her pen, give each dog a rawhide bone, sit down at Dan's desk. I've been thinking about his obituary, and I start writing it. I want to be sure it comes from me, no one else, and that it includes his canoeing the length of the Connecticut River, his chairing the zoning board, his full academic scholarship to Columbia. At one o'clock I realize I'm tired, that's why I'm not making any more headway on this, and I go to bed. I lie in the dark, my eyes open, my mind flooded with the details of his life. I'm nervous—I keep a hand on Lulu's flank, in back of my knees, and an arm encircling Cooper, up at my chest—but I'm not frightened. The next phase of my life has started, and with any luck it won't be any worse—any sadder or more horrifying—than this summer. In contrast, silence is a comfort, and darkness, peace.

Home Again

"We both have Monday off," says Maria, calling early on Thursday morning. "We could visit Dan, and help you with the yard."

I'm just up, making coffee, and again, I'm staring at the wood grain of the butcher-block counter. "I was going to call you, right away . . ."

"—Oh." Her second big, round *Oh*, like a gulp.

"I'm sorry," I say, stricken with guilt. "I got home late. I was going to call you before you went to work."

"Do you want me to come down today?"

I'd like her to move in for a month, but I say, "No, it's OK. I'm busy writing his obituary, and I'll be in and out, dealing with the funeral home. Monday's perfect."

"Did you call Dad?"

"—I didn't think they'd be up yet."

"I think they will be."

By calling them immediately Maria catches them as they're closing up the house, ready to make the two-hour drive to Hudson, to sit with Dan for a while in his hospice room.

I'm back at the desk, writing the obituary, when the phone rings again: Dr. Moore. Just calling to see how Dan is doing.

"All I wanted her to do was call me while he was alive," I growl to Margaret.

"Of course. But now that he's not her patient, it's safe."

In the afternoon, another call: Jenny, from hospice. This time I pick up the phone in the bedroom and stare out through the gritty porch at the unkempt yard, the dead peony heads drooping, unclipped.

"Mrs. Armitage gave him some morphine," I say, "the way you did. But it didn't help. His breathing never got any better."

Jenny pauses. She has Dan's chart in front of her, and hospice is about honesty; she has to go on. There is no record of Dan's receiving morphine last night.

Jenny fills my stunned silence with talk. Morphine is carefully regulated. One nurse must witness another's taking it, from a locked supply cabinet. The dosage must be precisely recorded: which patient, how much.

Mrs. Armitage isn't on duty today. Seems to me they should haul her in, but no, the nurse is allowed her time off. Jenny can't ask her about it until tomorrow, when Mrs. Armitage is back on the floor, leaving me to spend another twenty-four hours—daylight, dark, daylight again—periodically slammed with this.

I saw her give him the shot.

She didn't smile at us when she introduced herself.

I saw the syringe in her hand.

It held something else—liquid Tylenol, some placebo, she was indeed a monster, she decided it was best to let him go.

The funeral home is one of the grand, 19th-century houses in "uptown" Hudson, complete with a carriage portico under which I can park Lulu in the shade. The side door is always unlocked, though no one is ever in evidence. But if I wait a few minutes in the breathless silence of a house without air conditioning, in which windows are never opened, a pleasant woman—thin and pale, with dark hair that rests on her shoulders—will appear, as if she knew I was there. Once I see one of the young men who picked up Dan—the beefy, ruddy one—duck through a hallway. I begin to think of the woman, fondly, as Morticia, and the men—husband, brothers, in-laws, whatever they are—as the rest of the Addams family.

They need $325 in cash or check up front to initiate the cremation, so I use $300 of my office gift money. If I deliver the obituary by 4 p.m. today, Morticia tells me, she will get it into the local and Worcester papers tomorrow. I drop it off at 2 p.m. and it's published the next day. This feels like a miracle: people tell me what they'll do, and then they do it.

On Friday Jenny calls in the late morning. Mrs. Armitage has confirmed that she gave Dan morphine. By an oversight it was not noted in his chart; now it is. Confused and frightened once again, mightily tired of them, I choose to believe her.

And it's still not over. They've found Dan's toilet kit. When they moved him from the tiny room they forgot it, hanging on the bathroom doorknob, and I hadn't noticed it missing.

Jenny apologizes: "Our patients' belongings are important," she says.

It's important to me, too, that nothing, not one tiny shred of him, be left there. Even though once inside the hospital door, immediately I'm dropped into that life again, the smell a mix of antiseptic and deodorizer, the pale, ugly mustards and corals of another century, the shallow breathing of anxiety. Already I know where to stand at this elevator bank, and which car will come first.

The door to Jenny's office is open, but she's not there. The hunter green toilet kit—he was so pleased with it, another well-designed gadget, with all its different pockets, unfolding to reveal a hook on which it could be hung—sits on a table next to her desk. The hallway is empty; I don't know when she'll be back. So I enter someone else's space and take what I want. I'm standing in the hall, writing Jenny a note, when she reappears. We're polite. When Sam's wife, Juanita, was in hospice, Jenny became their friend. Maybe Juanita's medications were recorded correctly; maybe her things traveled with her. Or, maybe because they were friends, Juanita's care went well. I tell myself it doesn't matter, we didn't come here looking for a social life. But later, when people gush about how wonderful hospice is, I say, it's all right.

"Lulu, our lives have changed. We're going to Wal-Mart."

She doesn't object, even when I leave her in the car; she hops onto the back shelf and watches the action. It's the Saturday before school starts, and people smile at her, point her out to their children.

Inside, I buy a pint of Rustoleum, a brush, a roller, and a pan. I also find a dust buster, a smart chrome dish rack, and a clear rubber mat to go under it. All of these things are amazingly inexpensive.

When Maria and Jon come on Monday I ask them to paint the fuel tank; in half an hour, it's a glistening black. Jon hangs up the dust buster, and they help me move a few pieces of furniture to where I had always imagined them.

We eat lunch on the deck, and Maria says how strange it seems here without Dan. I agree because I fear she'd be shocked if I didn't, but for me, the summer stretched into forever, and he's been gone a long time.

They've brought Argos, their Lab, and we take the dogs for a walk around the old landfill where Dan used to run.

"Look!" says Jon. "A red-tailed hawk." We stop and watch the hawk glide on the wind over the grassy hill.

"Have you seen him before?" asks Maria.

"—I don't know. I haven't seen anything for months."

"Watch for him," she says, with a smile that's almost a wink, and I begin to see the red-tailed hawk. Once he soars over me as I work in the yard. Another time he follows me up our road as I drive home.

Women see Dan in their dreams that month. In Margaret's dream he wears his brown suede fedora and he smiles at her. From Santa Fe, Christi reports a happy dream: "We were both happy." Sonia e-mails to tell me that a graphic designer they worked with over the years, who sees the dead in her dreams, found herself with Dan. They were chatting away when she said, "Wait a minute—you can't talk."

"No," he said, "I'm fine."

I wish he would tell me this directly, but I have to take comfort where I can. Twice I dream about him. He's gone away on a trip and doesn't call. He's ill, in his hospital gown, bleeding from somewhere. His eyes are large black circles, Little Orphan Annie eyes. Unafraid, I reach for him. The dream ends.

The weekly Sunday service at the Zen Mountain Monastery is attended by the people in residence for the weekend retreat and anyone else who wants to come, and it's followed by lunch. When I arrive for my meeting with Sensei Shugen, the meal has just ended, and people are walking in groups toward the parking lot or hanging out together on the stone steps of the main building. This property first belonged to the Catholic Church, and a huge crucifix, with a life-sized Christ, still hangs high above the building's double doors. In contrast to the anguished Christ, the people below are all smiling, in a vaguely unsettling way. Their faces are kind and happy, but the uniformity of them makes me look for honesty, too. Not to mention that Dan disdained unremittingly cheerful people. Have I made another terrible mistake? What if he doesn't like it here?

Inside, a sweet young woman in a gray monk's robe finds Sensei Shugen for me. I'm late for our meeting—I didn't realize how far it was, how slow Sunday traffic would be—but he's patient with me. We sit on a bench at one of the long dining tables, and I start to relax. The severity of his shaved head is offset by the warmth in his eyes. Without hair to manipulate, all his beauty—his intelligence and compassion—comes through his eyes. That's true of all the men here, but especially of Shugen and of a taller, heavier man who's the cook and who remembers me when I visit later.

Shugen doesn't press me on whether Dan said the words "bury me, in the Zen Mountain Monastery." We're past that point; if I'm here today, then Dan is meant to be buried here. We work out some details for the funeral service, which will take place on Friday, September 13. If the Buddhists have no superstitions about that, then Dan and I don't either.

Only when we're finished do I have time to take my first look at the cemetery—and it's one of the most beautiful places I have ever been. A mix of deciduous and fir trees soars toward the sky. It smells like the pine needles underfoot. It's small, with headstones—about twenty—grouped here and there in clearings in the woods. The headstones are wooden plaques, two feet high and six inches across, curved at the top, with the name and dates of the deceased, nothing more, painted in black calligraphy. There's a stone bench, surrounded by the ferns he loved, between the cemetery and an outdoor worship site, and I sit there for a while. The woods are almost silent, with only a twitter, but in the distance I can hear a faint hum of traffic from the busy road I drove in on. This, too, is perfect: Buddhists are very much part of this world. I sit there, happy for the first time in months. He will love it here.

A week after Dan's discharge from Albany Medical Center I call Gloria, the patient representative, to say that we haven't received a departure questionnaire, and I would like one. She mails me a four-page questionnaire, and I fill it out carefully. It's multiple choice and not really intended for dissatisfied customers. There's no room for Dr. Gates of oncology or Dr. Slater of ethics, but I squeeze them in anyway. I make a copy for myself and send the original to Gloria with a note asking her to call me. When she doesn't call in a week, I call her. She's not available, so I leave a message.

In Provincetown with the dogs, I vow that I won't drive for a week, and I keep that promise. Renting a boat and driver to cast some of Dan's ashes into the sea at Long Beach proves impossible—the voyage would take a day and cost more than I can afford—so I relax and do the things that Dan always considered too hokey. I go on a whale watch and run back and forth on the ship with the others, laughing at ourselves, to see whales and dolphins. I take a literary walking tour of Provincetown, and outside the Unitarian church I am riveted by lines carved into a plaque on a bench:

They have only gone out ahead of us
and do not want to come home again.
We will find them on those heights up there
in the sunshine!
It is a beautiful day on those heights.

I use the verse on my Christmas card, and it consoles me every time I write it. A couple of people think I have lost my mind, but the rest understand.

Leaving the Cape, I stop at Long Beach and furtively cast some of Dan's ashes into the water and onto the dunes that soar thirty feet above the sea. It's a gorgeous September morning, on one of the most splendid beaches in the world. What a wonderful month he must be having, stretched out in the sun all day, indulging in fried clams at night.

Back home, I have a message from Dr. Singh's office, calling "to see how Dan is doing."

I try Gloria one more time, leave another message. She never responds. We've slipped off her screen. She doesn't need to deal with me anymore.

Instead, when I get home from work on a Monday in early October there's a message from Polly Naylor with her condolences. "The staff asked to be remembered to you," she says.

I join the church choir, and in that way get reacquainted with Audrey, who used to live down the road from us, and who, it turns out, attended the Neil Diamond concert in Albany.

"It was great!" she says, and then, reading my face, she puts an arm on my shoulders and gives me a squeeze. "He comes around all the time," she says. "We'll go next year."

In late October, unable to face Dr. Hahn, I find another doctor for myself. He's nice, taking some time to get to know me, and when I tell him about Dan, he sighs.

"Yeah, in my patients with lymphoma," he says, "by the time it's visible, it's pretty far along."

Click. Nine words, and everything's in focus.

By the time it's visible, it's pretty far along. All those words Dr. Moore spent on me without this simple, straightforward warning.

Two days before Thanksgiving, Paul has a stroke, sitting in a subway train on his way to work. He recovers and starts physical therapy to strengthen his left side. Finally, he stops smoking. "I'm going to play tennis again next spring," he tells me, and he does.

The Columbia classmate of Dan's who compiles information for the alumni magazine has a heart attack, and someone else makes sure that Bernie's remembrance of Dan gets into the magazine.

A coworker of Paul's, a man in his forties with two young children, is diagnosed with a brain tumor. Operable. We're all walking time bombs, he tells Paul.

In early December I return home from work to a phone message reminding Dan that he has an appointment with Kingston Neurology on Monday, December 9. I can't bear the idiocy of this, but I don't want to get charged for the appointment, so I call back. I tell the young woman who answers the phone that Dan has died; she asks me to hold. Soon another young woman answers, but she doesn't know why I'm calling, so I have to say the whole thing over again. She expresses her condolences, we hang up, and within half an hour, as I dreaded, Dr. Singh calls. Our conversation is brief. I was trying to reach that other doctor, she says, and I'm unable to say the words . . . *you should have . . . you shouldn't have . . .* they do him no good, his memory no honor.

In December the Anipryl that Cooper takes for his cognitive dysfunction stops working, and I get him an appointment with Dr. Tumulo, the head of the practice, who's known Cooper since he was a puppy. Dr. Tumulo says there's nothing more they can do for him; he's pleased the medication worked for so long.

On March 10, I sit in an examining room with Cooper in my lap, his head tucked under my arm. He's completely blind and almost completely disoriented. "Time for Dan to take care of Cooper again," Dr. Tumulo says gently, and I nod, unable to speak. Cooper doesn't even twitch at the shot; in half a minute he's gone. Dr. Tumulo leaves us, and I hold Cooper until he starts to cool. Then I lay him on the examining table as instructed, take off his collar, and kiss him good-bye.

I use Dr. Tumulo's words in an e-mail to friends.

"The celestial boulevard has never seen anything like those two," Paul writes back, and I'm comforted.

The holidays aren't sad so much as mysterious. To look at the photo taken by a helpful waiter the previous Thanksgiving, and to think that of the six of us—Jane, Judy, my mother, John—Dan, the youngest, would be missing just a year later, is incomprehensible.

At Christmas the choir is part of a group from church that sings carols in the Eden Park Nursing Home in Hudson. I make myself do this because I believe I should, no matter that none of the words I sing have anything to do with the Christmas of anyone living here. We walk through the halls, singing and ringing our bells, and finish our visit with a concert in the activity room, where three-dozen patients have been gathered. One woman reaches from her wheelchair for a little boy who's come with us, straining, yearning just to touch a child. Half of our audience has no reaction to our efforts. As I stand there, singing to people suffused with drugs or illness or both, I realize that Dan and I were lucky. He would have been miserable here. Yes, he had the massive misfortune to be struck down early by some combination of genetics and environment. The summer felt years long, but it wasn't; it was short, brutal, and merciful. He was spared this.

Easter. What did we do last Easter? I look in my daybook; Easter fell on March 31 last year, and we cleaned the road. That is, I came home from church at midday, wishing again that Dan would go there with me more than once a year, and I learned that he had devised a plan for picking up the litter along our road. The day was cool and cloudy, and I wanted to clean the daffodil beds, but I knew he was right—soon the trees would leaf out and the litter wouldn't be as visible. We walked our dogs on this road daily. We wanted it clean.

Dan put two black plastic trash bags into the trunk of my red Jetta. We took the dogs, since Dan took the dogs with him everywhere. I drove the two miles out our road to the Taconic State Parkway at about two miles per hour, pausing often. Dan walked behind the car, in paint-stained jeans, heavy work gloves, and a T-shirt plucked from the rag pile. Recyclables went into one bag, trash into another. Dan had run for 40 minutes that morning, and now he walked two miles out and two miles back, constantly bending and rising, picking up cans and bottles, cigarette packs and fast-food wrappers. It took about two hours, and during that time we saw a total of four cars—two going out, two coming back. We discussed the statistical implication of this: someone threw something out of the window of every car that ever drove down our road.

Back home I still had time to clean all our daffodil beds—back, front, and side yards—augment the soil with compost, and cover it with fresh mulch.

Dan showered and made popcorn—fresh kernels popped in vegetable oil, then salted. He sprinkled a few pieces onto the kitchen floor for the dogs and saved two cups for me to eat later. With the rest of it in a large bowl, he settled down in front of the TV to simultaneously read the Sunday *Times* and watch a golf match. For our Easter dinner, he fixed kielbasa. It was a perfectly normal Sunday.

CPSIA information can be obtained
at www.ICGtesting.com
Printed in the USA
BVHW051438080922
646450BV00005B/782